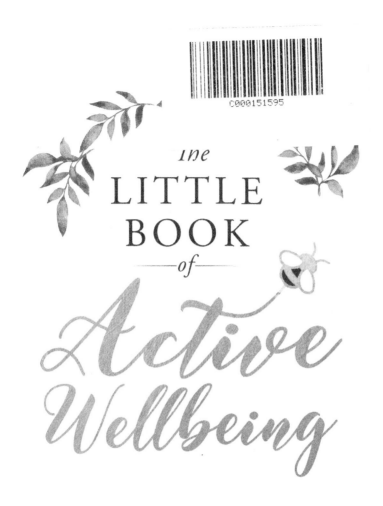

The
LITTLE
BOOK
of
Active
Wellbeing

MOVE MORE,
LIVE WELL

DIANE BROWN

Cover image by: Yesna99, 99Designs
Book design by: SWATT Books Ltd

Printed in the United Kingdom
First Printing, 2021

ISBN: 978-1-9168828-0-5 (Paperback)
ISBN: 978-1-9168828-1-2 (eBook)

FitBee Books
Thirsk, Yorkshire

www.fitbee.co.uk

To get started on your own journey to Active Wellbeing, discover the fabulous resources that complement this book at fitbee.co.uk/thelittlebook

Join my Active Wellbeing Community at facebook.com/groups/findtimefeelgood

Or follow me on Instagram @active_wellbeing_for_women

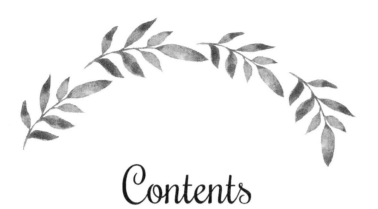

Contents

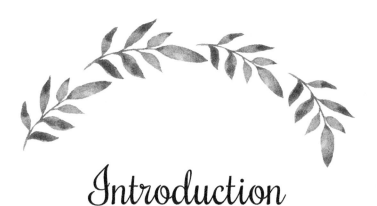

Introduction

$\mathcal{I}$ remember it like it was yesterday: the sheer sense of frustration, the sense of loss, and yet a deep, instinctive knowing that I had to do something.

Just 18 months earlier, I had been the fittest- and healthiest-ever version of myself, having recently completed a 17-hour ironman triathlon; the culmination of a dream that required four years of building up my strength and stamina, as well as generally getting my act together. I was so proud of my achievement, and it represented so much more to me than a fitness event. It symbolised a journey towards becoming the sort of person that I wanted to be – who I'd dreamed I could be.

I thought I would be fit and healthy for life; that I could finally be the kind of person who goes out and exercises just for the fun of it. From now on, I could join any event I wanted to at the drop of a hat. I'd finally made it, and nothing would ever be this hard ever again. Little did I know...

Is this book for you?

Having read the introduction, you may be thinking that this is the story of how I lost and then recovered my ironman fitness, and your reaction to that could be, *Well, this book isn't for me. There's no way I'd ever want to do an ironman event!*

Rest assured, that's not the story I'm here to tell, although I did lose my ironman levels of strength and stamina after becoming a mum, yes. This is the story of how I picked up the pieces and rebuilt my fitness anew, discovering a unique method for better living in the process, as I came to realise that there was a different way to approach exercise; a gentler, more self-compassionate way. A way that would help all women, but especially those at mid-life and beyond. Eventually, I gave it a name: Active Wellbeing.

This book is about how women struggling with fitness can finally feel in control of their own bodies, and why that matters.

But anyway, let's get back to the beginning...

Pregnancy hit me like a train. I felt sick, and I didn't want to move at all. Mid-pregnancy, I felt like I could exercise again, but at the same time, I was an anxious first-time mum. Which exercises was I 'allowed' to do? Was it safe? Should I be more careful, seeing as though I'd had three months off? Confusion led to inaction, and then my baby was here.

You see so many incredible stories of fit, athletic women who work hard to recover their fitness soon after childbirth. I am in complete admiration of them, but it wasn't my experience. My baby didn't let me sleep, ever. I was up all night, and then all through the days, too.

'Sleep when he sleeps,' they said.

Well, that advice doesn't work with babies who only ever want to be carried. Fear of him waking would prevent me putting him down, and fear of squashing him would stop me from sleeping myself. A sleep-deprived six months later, and I was not in good shape, neither physically nor mentally.

I'd worked so hard to improve my physical health, and now it felt like it was all just slipping away; like I'd gone into reverse, and all the work had been undone. I was back where I started, only worse, as I now had the family situation to balance, too. It was so frustrating. On the rare occasions where I had opportunities to exercise, I was either too tired or too busy being Mum to do anything, and so I started to wonder if it was time to accept frumpy mummy status, and consign my active lifestyle to the past.

No!

After many false starts and motivation struggles, I started to realise that it wasn't just my baby stopping me from exercising; something inside my head was getting in the way. I'd set out with a new plan and all the best intentions, but then either guilt or laziness would stop me putting my plan into action. That was when I started looking for help. I found a life coach, and decided to give it a try.

Just three sessions later, she had helped me to change my whole perspective on how to approach getting active again. I started to realise that it didn't have to be 'all or nothing;' it didn't matter if the plan wasn't carried out perfectly. Small steps and self-compassion were the ways forward. It took some years, and the road was a bumpy one at times, but I eventually went on to complete several more triathlons, a half-ironman and an ultramarathon in the proceeding years.

Now, this may be where you expect the 'happily ever after' story to end, but there's a twist to this tale.

Yes, I got back to ironman levels of fitness, but the funny thing about going back to something you once had is that it's never quite the same, and I soon realised that it wasn't really what I wanted, either. I'd been on a journey, climbing a mountain, crashing to the bottom and then climbing back up again, and although I loved the view at the top, I began to understand that maintaining such an intense level of training and commitment wasn't what I wanted anymore. I had learned the hard way that by pushing myself up those mountains again, I was only increasing my chances of crashing out and spending a few months (or years) doing not much at all. I began to wonder, *What if...* which is where the story of this book really begins.

What if there was a gentler, more balanced and more moderate way to approach fitness and exercise? *What if* you could enjoy being healthy and active without feeling you had to push yourself so hard? *What if* moving your body could be about developing a greater sense of wellbeing, instead of some weird modern-day penance for eating cake?

This is how the idea of Active Wellbeing was born.

This book is for women who want to find a better way to engage with fitness and exercise, but are not quite sure how.

It's for those who want to be more active, but have previously struggled with low motivation, lack of time and feelings of guilt for putting themselves first.

It's also for those who are generally active, but sometimes find themselves locked in an internal debate about whether or not it's self-indulgent to be taking care of themselves, forever asking if they're doing too much or if it's really worth the effort.

It's also for people who, like me, used to spend a lot of time on sport and fitness, but whose lives have now changed to the point that they need to find a new approach.

It's not about getting you fit for an ironman event or a triathlon; fitness doesn't have to look like that. You won't find much in this book about fitness plans or exercise routines. I am not a personal trainer. What you will find is a focus on health and wellbeing, and support in finding the right path for yourself. What's in these pages isn't just the sum of my own experiences, or what I've seen as a coach; it's grounded in psychological research. When I went back to university to study Sports and Exercise Psychology at the age of 42, I went there with the express intention of learning everything I could about the psychological factors that could help mid-life women to lead an active lifestyle, and to find evidence for mental wellbeing benefits that are so often mentioned anecdotally. What I discovered is that the worlds of personal anecdote and scientific evidence do indeed overlap, and I have made references to some of the most interesting research papers that I came across throughout this book.

At the end of each chapter, you will find short learning activities to help you explore your own thoughts and feelings about getting active, each designed to guide you along the small steps towards making Active Wellbeing a key part of your life.

The beauty of a book is that you can go at your own pace. Keep a pen or pencil handy for the written activities, and find yourself a lovely, quiet space to read (if all else fails, I find that locking myself in the bathroom works pretty well for at least five minutes).

I'm so happy you've chosen to let me help you on your journey towards Active Wellbeing, and I'm truly excited about what lies ahead for you.

Now, let's dive in.

CHAPTER ONE

Where Are You Now?

If you feel great about life right now, my guess is that you have probably picked up this book out of curiosity, or maybe even a desire to help others. If so, welcome! Part of living well is constantly looking for opportunities to adjust, nudge, grow and make life even better, so I hope you'll find lots of new ideas to put into practice. If, however, you feel like there should be more to life than what you are experiencing right now, and that something is wrong or missing, this book is aimed squarely at you.

As with any journey, to plan a route, you first need to work out where you are. There is a reason why you have picked up this book, and there's a reason why you have chosen to set aside some of your valuable time to read it. Those reasons will provide you with a foundation for making the changes that you want to see in your life, and so that's where we are going to start.

The difference between this and other 'fitness' books you may have read is that I am going to focus more on what's going on in your mind rather than your body. This means that you are going to have some thinking to do. I can't give you all of the answers, because YOU are the expert on your own life and your own thoughts, but I am going to guide you through a process that will help you uncover the path to an active lifestyle that works for you. This will require some work on your part, but first, let's take a quick look at where we want to end up. What is Active Wellbeing anyway?

Active Wellbeing in a nutshell

This whole book is about Active Wellbeing, so I don't want to open with too many spoilers! Still, it's helpful to know what we're aiming for.

If you imagine a Venn diagram (two overlapping circles), with 'moving your body' in one circle and 'feeling good' in the other, Active Wellbeing is where they overlap.

So, it's NOT about:

- setting elite sports targets
- being the best
- depriving yourself
- losing weight

It IS about:

- knowing what your body needs to feel good
- doing activities that fit in with your lifestyle
- looking after your own needs (as well as others' if relevant)
- owning your place in the world

We'll get into all of that in depth over the coming chapters, but for now, let's start with you.

Where Are You Now? check-in

It's great practice to check-in with how we are feeling on a regular basis, and to take a few moments to question our status quo and reconnect with ourselves.

This check-in is all about your wellbeing (note, not about your fitness). The purpose of this book is to learn how to work with our bodies in order to feel better. It's an important distinction, but we'll get into that more later.

Answer the following questions based on a typical week. If you don't often have a 'typical' week, base it on what you would consider your average (maybe not the best week, but not the worst, either):

1. How would you rate your current level of physical wellbeing? (1 = very poor, 10 = excellent)

2. How would you rate your current level of mental wellbeing? (1 = very poor, 10 = excellent)

3. How many minutes per week do you spend engaging in the following kinds of activity?

   a. Vigorous exercise (eg running, high-intensity workouts, spin classes, etc)

   b. Moderate physical activity (eg jogging, fast walking, dancing, swimming, cycling, very active job, etc)

   c. General / gentle physical activity (eg yoga, Pilates, gardening, walking, housework, active job, etc)

4. What changes to your physical activity routine would help you feel good?

Time for change?

Now that you've completed your first quick check-in, you'll have a sense of how happy you are with your current Active Wellbeing situation. It may be that you're feeling great, whatever the level of activity you're at, but for many of us, the thought of making a change is a welcome proposition. However, the truth is that effecting change is difficult. We're only human, after all.

Our brains are programmed to avoid change, and to highlight negatives before considering positives. As neuroscientist Rick Hanson says, 'The mind is like Velcro for negative experiences, and Teflon for positive ones.' This was great when we lived in the wild, and needed to stick to safe locations and scan for dangerous animals, but it is less helpful when we are consciously trying to make lifestyle changes in the modern world. If you've ever wondered why your brain seems to tell you to stay safely curled up on the couch, eating high-fat, high-sugar foods... well, you simply have your primitive brain to thank.

Luckily, we now have ways of quieting and overriding our primitive brains, but we need to do this consciously, at least to begin with.

Understanding your thought patterns

There's a well-known saying in the fitness world (it's written on the wall of the gym at my local leisure centre): 'What the mind believes, the body achieves.'

When we think about being active and getting fit, we have a natural tendency to focus on the body, whereas I find that focussing on the mind is far more helpful, especially when it comes to motivation. In this book, we'll be looking at your thoughts around exercise, while gently challenging some of the perceptions and beliefs you have about it.

So, let's take a look at where your thinking is currently...

What's getting in the way of you living the fit and healthy lifestyle that you'd love right now? (Circle all that apply)

1. You don't have enough time or energy.

2. You don't like how you look, or you feel like the fit bodies you see in adverts are unobtainable for you.

3. You're not an 'exercise-type' of person / you don't enjoy exercise.

4. You're too old to exercise.

5. You're too overweight to exercise.

6. You're too ill / injured to exercise.

7. Getting fit feels like such a huge, overwhelming task.

8. You're tired / stressed / overwhelmed / burnt-out by life.

9. You're bored / exhausted with goal setting.

Great work! Your answers will provide some really useful insights into what's been getting in your way, and here comes the good news, regardless of which answers you circled:

I'm going to help you deal with all of these thought obstacles.

My story

This book didn't exist when I needed it, which is why I am writing it now.

After the birth of my son, I felt like the whole world expected me to be happy, but I wasn't. Yes, I had gained a beautiful baby boy, but I had also lost something dear to me, a part of myself. Before pregnancy, I had been fit, healthy and able to spend my time as I pleased, and this wasn't something I'd always had. I had worked hard to get myself into a high-paying career, and equally difficult had been regaining fitness and health after losing the plot slightly in my twenties. So, to suddenly feel back at square one, or possibly even lower, was a difficult transition.

In addition to being sad and frustrated at the prospect of the mountain I would have to reclimb in order to recover my health and fitness, I also felt a loss of identity as I stopped spending time with work colleagues, dining at expensive restaurants and feeling important; instead spending my time at mum and baby groups, feeling ordinary and out of my depth.

I had never planned to feel ordinary; I wanted to go back to feeling like a woman in control. Yes, I knew in advance that my lifestyle would change, but I still wanted to be able to take part in exciting events, or at least feel well enough to be one of those active super-mums. You know, the ones in the adverts, who are happy and smiling while getting everything right for their kids, including being active outdoors and setting a great example of healthy living.

I had achieved great physical feats in the past, the pinnacle being Ironman UK in 2011, but now I had new barriers in the form of a lack of time and energy. I was totally exhausted from sleep deprivation, not to mention possible postnatal depression, which unfortunately my health visitor dismissed as not being serious enough for attention. However, despite these barriers, I knew I had to try.

I also knew my *why*. I needed to feel like myself again, not necessarily going back to the exact same lifestyle as before, but at least feeling as though I had some degree of control. I felt like I had gone from being somebody to just being somebody's mum, as my own needs, wants and desires seemed to have slipped off the radar. I knew that if I could just find a way to put some of my own priorities near the top of the pile – to value my own self-worth and do something just for me – it would help me feel more like my real self again.

That is why I turned to exercise, and ultimately to the concept of Active Wellbeing.

Why do you want to live a more active life?

Your reasons for wanting change may be different to mine, or they may be similar, but what's important is that it really matters to you, resonates with you and strikes an emotional chord that you can connect with as you power through the process. Looking great in a bikini is unlikely to be a strong enough *why*; joining a gym because your friend did is unlikely to be a strong enough *Why*.

Answer this question:

What really matters to **you**?

Strip everything down to the bare essentials, and think about what is most important in your life, now and for the future. Close the book for a minute, pick up a notebook and pen, or simply close your eyes and think. You are the expert in you, and you do have the answer to this. Once you find it, write it down.

If you feel you need a prompt, try filling in this sentence:

The most important thing in my life is .... because ....

That is your true starting point, your home and your centre. It's where you'll return to when life gets in your way. Keep it close.

Now, let's get back to confronting those thought obstacles, as you embark on your quest to boost and maintain your wellbeing...

The Seven Principles of Active Wellbeing

This book is all about learning how to understand your own thoughts in order to help you enjoy a more healthy, active lifestyle, because just like behaviours, our thinking can be habitual, too. You probably have many thoughts about exercise that have prevented you from living the active lifestyle you want, and it's these thought obstacles, which you identified earlier, that are standing in the way of the action you want to take. So, I am going to help you gently explore and challenge these ideas, and in their place, I offer you the Seven Principles of Active Wellbeing:

1. Put on your own oxygen mask first.

2. It's about how you feel (not how you look).

3. You were born to move.

4. You are good enough already.

5. Small steps are bigger than you think.

6. Connection is key.

7. It's about the journey, not the destination.

As we go on, we will address what each of these principles mean, why they are so important, and how you can put them to work in your own life.

At this point, you know where you stand, and you know how you feel about where you are with your own wellbeing, the good and bad. You know where you want to be, and, more importantly, you know why. You understand that this isn't just about attaining a different-shaped body or an arbitrary fitness goal. It goes much deeper than that.

You also know what's ahead of you in this book; the seven principles that will underpin your life and health. You know that this isn't purely about getting fitter, losing weight (*Bah humbug!* I have a lot to say on that, as you'll see) or being outdoors more because someone told you it was a good idea. It's about the very essence of living well.

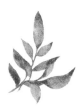

Ready to start?

Remember, in every chapter of this book, you will find a small task or activity to help move your thinking forward. In this chapter, you've had three tasks already, and in case you just read past them, like I often do, here they are again:

(Complete these tasks before moving on to the next chapter. It won't take long, and it will make all the difference. You're worth it!)

Time to write!

Where are you now? check-in

Answer the following questions based on a typical week. If you don't often have a 'typical' week, base it on what you would consider your average (maybe not the best week, but not the worst, either):

1. How would you rate your current level of physical wellbeing? (1 = very poor, 10 = excellent)

_____

2. How would you rate your current level of mental wellbeing? (1 = very poor, 10 = excellent)

_____

3. How many minutes per week do you spend engaging in the following kinds of activity?

a. Vigorous exercise (eg running, high-intensity workouts, spin classes, etc)

_____

b. Moderate physical activity (eg jogging, fast walking, dancing, swimming, cycling, very active job, etc)

_____

c. General / gentle physical activity (eg yoga, Pilates, gardening, walking, housework, active job, etc)

_____

4. What changes to your physical activity routine would help you feel good?

_____

_____

_____

_____

_____

_____

Understanding your thought patterns

What's getting in the way of you living the fit and healthy lifestyle that you'd love right now? (Circle all that apply)

1. You don't have enough time or energy.

2. You feel like the fit bodies you see in adverts are unobtainable for you.

3. You're not an 'exercise-type' of person / you don't enjoy exercise.

4. You're too old to exercise.

5. You're too overweight to exercise.

6. You're too ill / injured to exercise.

7. Getting fit feels like such a huge, overwhelming task.

8. You're tired / stressed / overwhelmed / burnt-out by life.

9. You're bored / exhausted with goal setting.

Why do you want to live a more active life?

Answer this question:

What really matters to *you*?

_____

_____

_____

_____

_____

_____

_____

_____

_____

_____

_____

_____

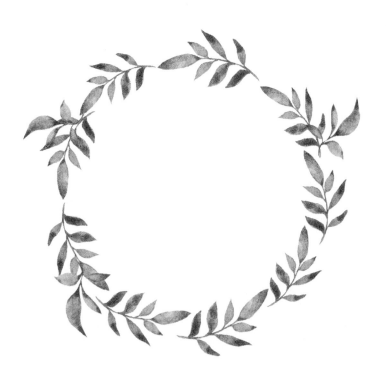

CHAPTER TWO

Put on Your Own Oxygen Mask First

Before I sat down to write this chapter, I went out for a run. When I got back, I made myself a drink and then took a nice hot shower. As I sit down, it is now 11:30am, and I have just half an hour of writing time before my next appointment. Given that this is officially my book-writing day, my decision to spend so much of my morning on myself instead of writing may seem surprising. Surely, I should have been glued to my desk since 5am, or nine at the very latest, maximising every last minute of the day?

If I had done this, would I have written more words? Possibly. Would they have been as effective in getting my message across? I seriously doubt it.

I know that my mind performs at its best, and is most productive, when I feel healthy and well, even more so immediately after a short burst of exercise. It's not simply my experience that tells me this; it is borne out in scientific studies, too. For example, in 2016, a review published in the *Journal of Science and Medicine* in Sport identified evidence of a positive link between physical activity and cognitive function.[1] In another paper, 30 adults were tested on their cognitive response to acute (short-burst) exercise, with the study confirming that general cognition was significantly improved in the period immediately following exercise, thus demonstrating that cognitive improvement is not simply an overall health effect,[2] but a direct daily benefit, too.

This effect doesn't only apply to my performance at work, but also to my performance in life, including everything that my brain has an influence on. It certainly applies to my ability to take care of others in my life from a place of calm and wellbeing.

Exercise can even help improve our emotional resilience, particularly for women in mid-life, where it's been suggested that physical activity may help us to cope with menopausal symptoms through increased 'coping efficacy' on a day-to-day basis.[3]

If you're a woman reading this book, you may feel that other people's needs take up most of your time. For some people, even taking a moment to read a book feels like an indulgence, but it's really not. You, like your children, your spouse, your relatives and your neighbours, are a person in your own right, and you deserve to have your own needs met, too.

There are also women for whom the demands on their time are much less – perhaps the responsibilities of childcare and work have now passed – and yet the impact of all those previous outpourings of energy remain. It's common for such women to feel disconnected from their own identity after giving so much of themselves in the service of others, with the realisation of this coming at different times. Everyone's lives are different; we each have a unique patchwork of people around us who we feel the need to support and nurture. Sometimes, this need comes from a simple desire to help others, while at other times it can feel like a duty or obligation.

The people we need to help could be children, elderly parents, sick relatives, clients or even colleagues at work. It is known that women who have children are less likely to participate in physical activity compared with women who do not, a phenomena that prompted a 2005 study involving 12 mothers of young children from a variety of societal backgrounds and economic statuses. Here, it was found that the 'ethic of care' was an important factor in determining the ability of women to take up regular physical activity,[4] and it is this inbuilt sense of responsibility for taking care of others that prevents many women from taking care of their own needs, including the need for physical activity and exercise.

Pause for a moment, and reflect on all the pulls on your time that come from other people. In your notebook, make a list of all the things you do for others, and who you do them for. Read it back to yourself. It may not be a short list.

Many women unconsciously pick up more and more people to try to help as they go through life.

'Yes, but I enjoy supporting others, and they're counting on me!' you may exclaim.

That's absolutely fine, and I'm not suggesting that you stop doing things that you enjoy and love. What I am suggesting is that you look at how your own needs are being met, and ask yourself if this is impacting all of those people you strive to support. If you can be responsible for others, there's no reason why you can't be responsible for yourself, too.

What are your needs?

You need to be your own number one priority. If you don't take care of yourself, you could eventually end up in a position where you are unable to take care of anyone else. Maybe this has happened to you already; maybe it has happened to someone you know. It definitely happened to me.

This is why they tell aeroplane passengers to put their own oxygen masks on first before helping anyone else, including children. Does it seem selfish? Would you feel guilty? Maybe, but you do it because you know it's the best way to help.

We've been brought up in a culture where many expectations are placed on women, sometimes without our even being aware of it. Women are expected to 'do it all,' mothers are expected to 'always be there for the kids,' and daughters are expected to be the 'responsible' ones more so than sons. These cultural expectations sink into our subconscious to such an extent that even the most self-aware of us can be caught feeling guilty about going for a run instead of taking the kids to the park, or leaving work on time to hit the gym. How would you view the choice of visiting an elderly relative versus going for a social bike ride with friends? We may be drawn to the latter, perhaps being in desperate need of a break, but we feel a sense of shame about it because our social programming tells us that looking after the elderly relative is the caring and responsible thing to do.

Let's take a step back and look at the bigger picture.

Your mental health and wellbeing are dependent on you taking care of yourself, which means that all those other people who you nurture and support depend on you having good mental health and wellbeing, too. With this in mind, it makes sense that the best way for you to help the people around you is to take care of yourself first and foremost, enabling you to radiate positive energy that will flow into their lives. Also, consider this:

When the people you care about see how much importance you place on your own self-care, you act as a role model, showing them that they can do the same. Whether it's children, friends, colleagues or older relatives, it's part of human nature to look around at what everyone else is doing; this is how a culture is built. When you take a stand and resolve to look after yourself, you will inspire others to do the same, and the ripple effect can be phenomenal. This ripple effect also extends beyond the human population and into the broader ecosystem, too. Healthy, thriving, happy people are better equipped to view the world in a positive light, appreciate the value of their surroundings and feel more connected to both the world and their fellow humans, all of which goes a long way towards forming a lasting basis for building a more sustainable and healthy future for everyone.

Whatever your past experiences, you can always start again from today. The human body is incredibly resilient, and capable of great feats of healing when given the chance.

A sense of freedom

Autonomy, or to put it in more common language, 'a sense of freedom,' is an important component of wellbeing, and it also turns out that a sense of freedom is one of the benefits that women gain from being active.

In 2010, a study was conducted on attendees at an Active Women's Festival,[5] where women were given the opportunity to try out a range of different physical activities. Afterwards, participants reported that they gained more 'headspace,' increased opportunities to 'do their own thing' and to 'get some of their life back.' This was from just a weekend-long festival, so imagine what being able to spend months enjoying your activities of choice would feel like!

Similarly, a further study in 2016 examined how 18 mothers with young children resisted the expectations of motherhood to engage in more physical activity.[6] The interviewed mothers frequently referred to experiencing 'mother guilt' and feeling 'selfish' when they first tried to make time for being active. However, once they got going, the women reported being able to use exercise to 'feel good,' 'create a space for relaxation,' and 'reconnect with their self-identity.'

Making it happen

OK, let's say you're with me so far. You understand that you need to take care of yourself, and that you need to put yourself higher on your own list of priorities. You also realise that being more active would be great for your mental health and wellbeing.

BUT...

'I haven't got enough time!'

You may genuinely feel as though you can't physically get away to exercise, or believe that the stress of trying to fit another thing into your busy schedule would be counterproductive. Well, I'm here to tell you that part of the solution to this is a change in mindset.

I'm aware that being told how the solution to lack of time is mindset could make some people very angry, so before you throw the book across the room, let's just put that to one side for the moment while we take a look at some of the practical issues around time.

Many people believe that if they don't have time to go to the gym or attend a fitness class, it means exercise isn't for them, but that just isn't the case. There are many ways to exercise and stay active; after all, it's really just moving your body around at different speeds and in different directions, and movement is exactly what our bodies were designed for.

Exercise and parenting

One of the most common barriers to women getting more exercise is not being able to get time away from children, but while this isn't ideal for developing that sense of autonomy, the great thing about being around kids is that they love to move. You would be surprised at the many types of exercise you can do these days that make it easy for kids to watch or join in (eg dancing, aerobics, hula-hoop, piggy backs and YouTube yoga).

There are lots of ways to be energetic at home; all it takes is a bit of imagination, planning and open-mindedness about what counts as exercise. For me, one of the positives that came from the 2020 Lockdown experience was how it helped to make us much more creative about being active with kids, as we searched for new things to try. I even found my husband skipping in the back garden during play time one afternoon!

Another great way to get active with the kids is to encourage them to have more outdoor time. Research into Forest Schools,[7] where children spend much of their time outdoors, showed improvements in confidence, motivation and concentration, as well as language, communication and physical skills.

Any action that increases your children's outdoor time will be hugely beneficial, both for them and for you.

Turn everyday tasks into movement opportunities

Another way to get moving is to incorporate it into your everyday routine. Let's take housework for example (not that I'm suggesting housework is your responsibility any more than it's anyone else's, of course). Rather than viewing the chores as a necessary evil, look at where you can inject more movement. Speed walk around the house, race the kids to see who can put the clothes away the fastest, go up and down the stairs more times than you really need to, and wiggle your hips to the music while washing up. What you do doesn't really matter, as long as you try to do it at a brisk pace and with more movement. Do at least 20 minutes of housework in this way, and make sure that you count it as being active, recognising the extra effort you have made to take care of yourself. Notice how this makes you feel, and then make plans to repeat the process the following day.

It doesn't have to be housework if that's not your cup of tea (it's certainly not mine); the point is simply to find ways to include more vigorous movements in your daily routine, whatever that looks like. Take the stairs rather than the lift at work, march on the spot while waiting for the kettle to boil, use your lunch break to have a walk, and order your coffee to go and then catch up with a friend as you walk. Get creative about incorporating more movement into everything you do.

Focus on energy, not time

Another important feature of creating time for exercise is not thinking about time at all. I know that sounds strange, but when we feel tired and we don't have time for exercise, the issue is very rarely time management. It's more often a case of energy management.

Think about it. When is the last time you said, 'I don't have time to go out to buy chocolate bars,' or 'I don't have time to sit down and drink a cup of tea,' or 'I don't have time to order a pizza?' If you are the proud owner of a young baby, I will allow an exception here (I drank cold tea for at least the first 10 months), but for everyone else, notice how you manage to find time for the things you really want to do, particularly when you believe that they will give you a much-needed energy boost.

Exercise feels harder because although we know that it helps improve energy levels, we first need to expend some energy before reaping the rewards, and this can seem like a big hurdle. However, once we get started with small amounts of activity, we begin to experience improved sleep and raised energy levels, which allows us to increase our activity levels, which leads to further sleep improvement and perhaps a desire to eat better, which increases our energy levels further, thereby creating a virtuous upward spiral.

So, how do we get started?

Have you noticed that there are certain times of the day where your energy is either high or low? Even if you feel tired most of the time, are there times of the day where you feel a little less tired than others? If you're not sure, try monitoring your fluctuating energy levels over the next few days, and make a note of what you find.

Once you become aware of your energetic rhythms, you can begin to work with them by adding movement into the parts of the day where your energy is higher. Planning to be more active when you feel a bit less tired will help you gain energy that can be then be fed into other parts of the day.

Feel good about whatever you achieve, and remember that small steps in the beginning are not only OK, they're also the best approach to sustainable, long-lasting change. We'll go into this in more detail later in the book.

Find what feels good

Notice the types of activities you're more attracted to doing. Notice what makes you feel energised, and what makes you feel tired. Notice the difference between physical tiredness (the heavy feeling in your body) and mental tiredness (the heavy feeling in your head). It can feel great to be physically tired at the end of the day, which often leads to a good night's sleep, but mental tiredness from the moment of waking is likely a sign that something's not quite right.

Maybe you dread the school run, and find the whole routine an onerous challenge, but setting aside 10 minutes for yoga early in the mornings may give you a boost that lets you feel more awake. The same principle applies to any 10-minute burst of activity, as we all need breaks from our work in order to freshen up and be more productive. A brief flurry of movement will add to our productivity, not damage it, which is why energy management is so much more important than time management.

Whatever your situation, the most important step is finding a physical activity that you enjoy, and if you don't know what that could be yet, try new things. If you're stuck in a rut, try new things. If you're feeling adventurous, try new things...

I think you get the idea.

Remember, just because you've tried a certain class or gym in the past and not liked it, this doesn't mean that you're not an 'exercise person,' and neither does the fact that you hated PE at school, or were told you weren't good at it. And while we're at it, being a particular age, shape or size does not mean that you are not an exercise person, either.

What is an exercise person anyway? An Olympian, or one of those men you saw jogging in town last week, or someone who gets up at 5am every day to go to the gym? I'm not any of those people, but I can still move my body and be active, and so can you.

A note on menopause and perimenopause

A really important transition stage in a woman's life is menopause, and also the perimenopause stage leading up to it. Luckily, menopause is shaking off its taboo status, and now more women, employers and medical professionals are giving it the attention it deserves.

Although this shift in hormones affects people differently, it is well known that many women struggle with it both emotionally and physically. Menopausal symptoms can include low energy, anxiety and depression, and while exercise is not a magic wand that will resolve these issues, research suggests that it does help to manage them, and thus to improve women's quality of life. In a study of 164 mid-life women with previously low-activity levels, researchers followed the participants' progress throughout a four-month programme that was split into three groups: walking, yoga and control (ie no change), where it was found that in both the yoga and walking groups, mood, quality of life and mental health all improved.[8]

In 2020, the journal *Menopause* published a study examining more than 70 different walking programmes, which reported a 91% success rate for improving at least one menopause-related medical issue before concluding:

> *'Further research would be recommended to establish the therapeutic value of walking programs for women with specific focus on typical menopause symptoms at different stages of menopause.'* [9]

I say, 'Let's not wait around for further studies. Let's get moving now!'

My message to menopausal women everywhere is don't overlook the remedies at your doorstep. Exercise isn't a cure, but then menopause isn't an illness, and a more active lifestyle leads to a better-functioning body, which in turn leads to an easing of difficult symptoms. So, if you're in the midst of menopause or perimenopause, this book is definitely for you.

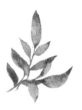

Ready to put yourself first?

For many women, putting themselves first will feel like an unusual, perhaps even indulgent, concept, but the fact is that you must! As I've explained in this chapter, we can only give our best to our loved ones if we take care of ourselves first. It isn't selfish to consider our own health and wellbeing needs, it's actually the most responsible and caring thing we can do. It also makes us role models of healthy behaviour to those around us, creating a positive ripple effect.

So, before you do anything else, remember to put on your own oxygen mask first!

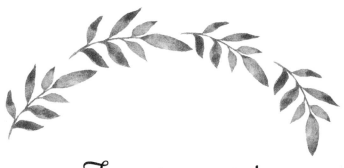

Time to write!

1. In your notebook, divide a page into two columns. In the first, list all the needs that you have in your life.

   (You could start simple, with things like food and water, but try to go beyond that. What do you really need to support your wellbeing? Think about what brings you happiness, fulfilment and relaxation, in addition to meeting your basic needs.)

   In the second column, make notes and comments on how, or if, each need is being met.

2. Reflect on what you wrote. If you can see a change you want to make, note it down.

3. List three things you could do differently if you started putting yourself first.

4. Consider how these changes could benefit your loved ones.

CHAPTER THREE

It's About How You Feel, Not How You Look

I find myself writing this chapter during the first COVID-19 Lockdown of 2020. It's been around six weeks since the government first ruled that we should only leave the house for shopping essentials and our daily exercise. How long will this Lockdown continue? Well, you are more likely to know the answer to that than I am right now, but I can say that in just six short weeks, we have begun to learn some new and interesting things about the world, ourselves and the role of exercise.

Before COVID-19, I was already passionate about getting the message across that exercise is about how you feel, not how you look. Sadly, the fitness industry remains dominated by weight-loss adverts, beach body quick-fixes and young women in unnecessarily tight and revealing gym wear, but this didn't stop a quietly growing movement of people from realising that they wanted to exercise because it helped them feel good. These people could often be found at yoga classes, local park runs and occasionally out cycling on sunny afternoons, as gentler, 'just for fun' activities gained in popularity, largely due to their non-competitive and inclusive nature that said anyone could participate.

Unfortunately, even with these great (and often free) options available, a large number of people still felt that exercise wasn't for them, and maybe you were one of them. The issue here is predominantly a result of self-identification; 'I'm just not an exercise-type of person,' is a phrase I hear a lot, and it is usually associated with a person's feelings about their looks, their size or their physical abilities, not to mention the crushing fear of, 'What if people see me try and fail? I'll be so embarrassed. I'll look ridiculous.'

During the initial COVID-19 outbreak, a survey conducted by Sport England reported that 63% of people felt that exercise was more important during Lockdown than it had been previously. This is a fascinating discovery, and it's worth taking some time to unpack.

What was it that made people feel like exercise had become more important? Here's a multiple-choice quiz, so let's see if you can find the answer:

Why did 63% of people think that exercise was more important during COVID-19 than it was pre-Lockdown?

- **a.** Because they needed to get beach-body-ready to sunbathe in the back garden.

- **b.** Because they thought that a global pandemic would be great time to try to shed a few pounds

- **c.** Because they had a Zoom party coming up and nothing new to wear, so needed to squeeze back into an old party dress.

OK, I think you maybe get my point. I suspect that none of these were the case for most of the respondents. If their experience of Lockdown was anything like mine, or yours, they probably noticed that getting exercise helped them feel better. There was also a realisation for many that keeping a fit, healthy body makes a real-life difference when it comes to fighting off illness. This is something we knew already, but COVID brought it closer to home, as even the very fact that daily exercise was permitted and seen as an essential activity speaks to its ability to helps us feel better, mentally as well as physically.

We may never get beach-body-ready or back into that old party dress, but it doesn't matter because those are not the truly important things in life. Besides, we'll be too busy feeling good to even notice.

The fitness ripple effect

In this chapter, I'll further explore the role of exercise, discussing how it makes us feel and explaining the ripple effect that it can have on the rest of our lives.

The scientific community has long agreed that mental and physical health are linked, and when we see this presented in simple terms, we may wonder why we needed science to spell it out for us. After all, the brain is part of the body, so it stands to reason that a healthy brain is needed for physical as well as mental health. Our physical bodies wouldn't be in a great state if our brains failed to do their job of running the show.

We are whole beings – living organisms with everything interconnected – and so to a large extent, physical and mental health are one and the same. The separation only came about historically to allow scientists and philosophers to specialise in specific areas, and now modern research is bringing home the message that we can't separate the two any longer. This demonstrates the necessity for a more holistic approach; there is no point in driving ourselves to physical perfection if we damage ourselves mentally in the process, which, sadly, is the path that the fitness industry often take us down (sometimes deliberately).

The dangers of an image-focussed approach to exercise

Here's where I get angry about the fitness industry's obsession with looks, so strap yourself in!

First of all, focussing on how we look is likely to bring us down. This shouldn't be the case, but unfortunately, there is a lot of money to be made by telling women that they don't look quite right, or could perhaps look better. This is how marketing works; to create a demand for a product, you point out a problem and then offer the solution. Thus, what could have been, 'Come and join our dance class and have some fun,' becomes, 'Feeling like you need to shed some Christmas pounds? Join our dance class for fast slimming results.'

Now, let me be clear. The only reason this type of marketing works is because many of us have become too focussed on how we look, often to the detriment of how we feel. Meanwhile, the money keeps pouring in, making it profitable to keep it that way.

I'd like to believe that maybe the tide is starting to turn, though. A promising sign is that when I recently introduced myself at a training workshop, and explained that I was interested in fitness for feeling good above looking good, I received a spontaneous round of applause. This tells me that many women are sick of being told how to look and what to do, and just want to feel healthy and happy. That's a far more empowered mindset to bring to your body than what's being sold by marketing executives.

Another pitfall of the diet world is its focus on week-to-week results. Nurturing wellbeing is a long-term commitment fraught with inevitable ups and downs, and so a realistic, compassionate approach is always going to be far more sustainable than an expectation of bigger and better results on a weekly basis.

We are not machines. You can't simply programme the body to lose fat or gain muscle on a set schedule; we are more complex than that. We live real, messy lives. It is whole wellbeing that enhances our lives, not chore-like routines or a set of meaningless goals to hit.

Worrying about how we look can sometimes stop us before we even get started. I'm often saddened by the women who feel they can't begin to exercise until they've lost some weight, as while it's true that some people may need to take a more careful approach than others, there is always an appropriate activity that we can do relative to our respective starting points.

Real health and wellbeing is about looking after yourself, not what other people think, and whatever our size or shape, we all have a right to self-care. Waiting only wastes time, which in turn prolongs the experience of feeling bad about yourself when you could be taking manageable steps towards looking after your body (and your mind) instead.

As we begin to move our bodies, we feel ourselves becoming stronger, and our mental health, confidence and self-esteem increase along with it.[10] Even moderate amounts of physical activity have been shown to help improve mental health,[11] which is why the best type of beginner's exercise is always something gentle. This initial success will deliver a much-needed confidence boost to your subconscious, and allow you to build up over time. We cannot allow insecurities about how we look to get in the way of this process.

Doing something – anything – is a powerful first step. It reminds you that you are in charge of your own destiny, enabling a mindset that will have a ripple effect across the rest of your life.

Get outdoors

We can really turbo-charge the feel-good part of exercise by taking it outdoors. Most people recognise how much better they feel after being outdoors for a while, even during 'bad' weather, as there comes a great sense of connection to nature, followed by a lovely snug feeling of warmth when we eventually return home.

Evidence pointing to the advantages of spending time outdoors and around nature is increasing all the time, with researchers identifying mental health benefits such as lowered stress levels, reduction in depression and anxiety, and improved cognitive function.[12,13] Combine this time outdoors with some gentle-to-moderate movement, and you will fortify your gains.

So, next time you feel low, anxious or stressed, try taking a walk outside, and if you've got kids, encourage them to go with you. The whole family benefits from spending as much time outdoors as possible, and although it's not always easy to coax children out of the house – trust me, I know all about this – there are strategies that can help (for tips and ideas, check out the resources available at fitbee.co.uk/thelittlebook).

Mindfulness and movement

As mentioned earlier, I am writing this as we adapt to the global presence of COVID-19, which I think has really brought home the importance of being in the present moment for a lot of people. When we experience dramatic changes to our daily routines, to the point where we genuinely fear for our futures, an appreciation of the present moment – not to mention the number of present moments we may actually have left – takes on a much greater significance.

When our heads are no longer filled with to-do lists, future plans and past mishaps, we finally begin to notice the current world as it is now. Even during dark times, the world around us is amazing and full of opportunities, but only if we choose to see them. Our lives are created in the now.

This is a subject that the great philosopher Eckhart Tolle speaks about at length during public speaking engagements, as well as in his books. We do not create our futures in the future, we create them now. Now is the only time we have available to make decisions and take action,[14] and learning to be present in the now will help us to make better decisions and take better actions.

Physical activity can be a great device for bringing a wandering mind into the present moment. I was once asked if I got bored during a 17-hour ironman I had just completed, and my reply was that I couldn't get bored because there was far too much to think about. During each and every second of the event, I had to concentrate on what I was doing in that moment in order to get the best result. I was completely absorbed and completely present.

Fortunately, you don't need to complete an ironman to experience living in the present moment. In fact, you can even practice without the exercise part. Some great activities to help you feel grounded are simple ones that require your hands, like baking, gardening and mindful colouring or drawing, but really any activity that absorbs your attention and forces you to concentrate on the world outside your own head will be of help. When I tried explaining mindfulness to my husband, he told me that it sounded like what he does while riding his motorbike, and I'd have to agree that this does seem to be a sufficiently absorbing activity where being present in the moment is key.

Can you think of any others?

Yoga often comes up on these lists, as it's a great blend of mindfulness and movement – one that I absolutely love – and there are many others that fall into this category, such as mindful walking, mindful running and mindful swimming.

What examples can you think of?

Being active can help you feel free

Another great benefit of physical activity is the sense of freedom it can give us. If you've ever enjoyed the sensation of the wind against your face as you freewheel a bicycle downhill, you'll know exactly what I mean. Being outdoors among the elements brings a wonderful sense of freedom, and for women escaping household chores and hours of childcare, that sense of freedom can be very literal, too.

In a world rife with external circumstances beyond our control, it's common to feel trapped and powerless, but getting active outside helps to remind us of our own place in the universe, and how we are part of nature and free to choose our own paths in life.

Who knows what would happen if more women realised this!

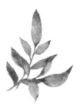

Ready to feel good?

For too long, the fitness industry has been dominated by the idea that it's all about looking good, and this has had a deeply damaging effect on many women. It's an idea that plays into the hands of marketing executives and their cheap tactics that rely on 'sexy' images, but as far as our health and wellbeing goes, it completely misses the point.

Being fit and active is about feeling good, and while this may not be an ideal pitch for a magazine ad, it is nevertheless a far more important and worthwhile goal.

I would love for you to explore physical activity with a focus on feeling good, as you play around with different activities until you find the ones that are most fun for you.

Oh, and if you still want to be beach-body-ready, just head straight for the beach, because you ARE ready!

Time to write!

For this activity, you will need to set aside 20 minutes and have a pen and notebook handy. Don't just skip over this part – do it! It will be worth it.

1. Write a list of all the activities you enjoyed as a child. Include games played, places visited and people involved.

2. Reading back over your answer, can you see any common themes in the activities you most enjoyed?

3. Looking at your current lifestyle, where and how could you add more of these enjoyable themes?

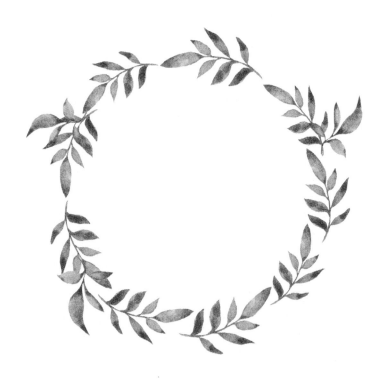

CHAPTER FOUR

You Were Born to Move

Humans have been responsible for an enormous number of technological advancements over the past 200 years. Where once we might have farmed the land or joined the daily grind of factory work, many of us now spend much of our working days sitting at a computer desk. Machinery and automation have taken over all but the most highly skilled of manual tasks, in a relentless pursuit of efficiency and productivity that has greatly reduced the necessity to move our bodies, instead increasing the demands on our brains.

Even our leisure time has become automated, with social media, SMART TVs and computer games dominating our free time, and during the first COVID-19 Lockdown of 2020 (still happening as I write), we couldn't even go out to meet up with friends, forcing us to rely on technology for our interactions. All of this combines to reduce how much time we spend outside, experiencing the world around us and moving our bodies.

That, as they say, is 'progress' for you.

The resulting impact of these changes to society could be a whole book in and of itself (and probably is), but for now I only want to focus on the impact it has had on our physical activity. It has deprived us of access to one of the most fundamental ingredients to our health and wellbeing: movement.

How did fitness become separated from living?

There is a reason why the fitness industry is a quite modern phenomenon, only really developing in the past 100 years. Try telling a 17th century farmer that he needs to do a HIIT workout, for example. He'd think you were mad. For thousands of years, we had to move to survive, and we are hard-wired for energy conservation because of this.

Seeking out ways to expend less energy isn't a personality flaw, it's a deeply ingrained survival instinct, but as we've learned to develop tools and machinery to do the heavy lifting for us, this instinct has led us to the lack of movement seen across society today.

You don't have to look far for evidence of the luxury status that our culture assigns to 'doing nothing,' be it all-inclusive holidays, spa day retreats or cinemas where the size of the seats increases based on the cost of a ticket. The message is clear, and it's all around us: 'If you can afford to sit still, you have achieved success,' hence a sedentary life becoming a desirable one. Combine this with physically demanding work being associated with a lack of skills, and thus being valued less in terms of both wages and social status (how much less paid and respected are care workers or cleaning staff in comparison to bankers or marketing consultants?), and you have a recipe for us not moving very much at all.

What has this done to our perceptions of sport and exercise? Well, certainly there is a prevailing notion that it must be 'hard work,' a view frequently pedalled by personal trainers and coaches from the school of 'no pain, no gain' (luckily, they're not all like that). There's also the issue of image, and what 'we' as the general public think that 'they,' the sporty, athletic types, are really like. I often hear assumptions made about people who exercise regularly being naturally fit and finding exercise easy, not to mention the many women who associate sport with sweatiness, unattractiveness and even embarrassment.

Commercial interests have focussed the purpose of women's fitness on looks and appearance, promoting portrayals of super-slim women with immaculate hair and skin, who could probably wear a bin bag and still look great according to Western beauty ideals. The quick sell here is 'join this gym' or 'buy this product,' and you, too, can look like this. Of course, the featured women in these ads often look that way thanks to strict regimens, genetic attributes or by sheer virtue of youth. Whatever the case, they certainly didn't join that gym and magically transform in the space of a few weeks.

When we buy into the idea that exercise is about making us look a certain way, we leave ourselves open to rapidly becoming disheartened if we don't see immediate results.

Similarly, if our experience at the gym is at odds with what we'd hoped for, we tend to flee and never return, creating a situation that reinforces the sense of 'us' and 'them' in our minds, with 'us' being the real-life, ordinary woman, and 'them' the unattainably attractive and super fit.

Women who are unable to identify with the type of person who fits the exercise stereotype will often find it very difficult to motivate themselves to pursue physical health. Where has this stereotype come from? Not from our bodies, which are designed and built for movement, but from our minds, and the cultural messages that we have been fed.

The biggest irony in all of this is that we are all 'naturally fit' because we are all born to move, and the real truth about exercise is that anyone can do it. You don't need to be a certain type of person, and you definitely don't need a certain kind of skill or ability. In fact, I would suggest that the less ability you have the better, as learning something new adds to the fun of it.

What types of activity really count when it comes to movement and fitness? Honestly, anything. We tend to think in terms of formally organised activities when it comes to fitness, as PE at school later gives way to exercise classes, with maybe some yoga, swimming or a gym membership on top. While these are all great activities to try (and an organised, supportive environment can be helpful for many), they are certainly not the only kinds of physical activity that count.

There are many different ways to move your body more. The most important thing is to find what you enjoy, as ultimately these are the activities where motivation is easiest. Could you include any of the following in your daily routine: dancing, walking, hula-hooping, roller skating, playing tig (AKA tag), skipping, trampolining or gardening? If any of these sound more appealing than whatever you're trying now, it's worth giving them a go. Your body will appreciate you for it.

Finally, exercise does not have to be hard work, despite what the 'no pain, no gain' types would have you believe. It can be fun, and it doesn't have to be an add-on to your day; it can be part of how you live your life. Taking a 20-minute walk during a lunch break can become your new normal. Cycling to work or to the shops a couple of times a week can become your new normal. Choosing to meet a friend for a swim, rather than having a glass of wine in the pub, can be your new normal.

The above are just a handful of examples of choices that could help you feel fitter and happier as you live your everyday life.

Next, we'll look at more ways to get moving.

Moving is your birthright; reclaim it

You are entitled to move, simply by virtue of being human; you don't need anyone's permission, nor do you need lots of money to be more active. Buying fancy gear and paying for classes can be fun, but they're not necessary. Walking, for example, is a great exercise that can be started for the price of a decent pair of shoes. You can also find loads of free workout and dance videos on YouTube, with endless options to prevent you from getting bored. From HIIT workouts to yoga, there is something to suit every level of fitness.

If you have kids in tow, how about trips to the park? A football kick around or a frisbee game is good for both you and them, and now that we're thinking about it, when was the last time you played a game of rounders? (No, I could never hit the ball, either!) The point isn't to be a great sportsperson, but simply to get moving and have fun.

Many women feel like they don't have enough time to fit in exercise (as talked about in Chapter Three), but there are several ways to tackle that. Mindset is certainly a consideration, as we've seen, and there are practical strategies, too. Let's say that the target is to do 30 minutes of exercise in a day. This could be broken down several ways, eg:

- 2 x 15 minutes of fast walking (useful if there's somewhere you need to go anyway)
- 3 x 10 minutes playing with the kids (good for young children. If you can't beat them, join them)
- 6 x 5 minutes skipping (if you're at home throughout the day, this helps to make sure that you take some breaks from other tasks)
- 10 x 3 minutes dancing to music while the tea brews (I know this sounds like a lot of tea, but it's about right for me!)

One way to find more time is to replace a habit that you know doesn't help you with a movement one. For example, what if every time you reached for your phone, you did some yoga stretches or ran on the spot for a minute instead? I know that for a lot of us, this would lead to our movement rate skyrocketing!

Of course, you can pick and mix, mix and match, and add your own ideas. Find a format that works for you (it may look different on different days), and you'll find that the options are almost limitless.

But what counts?

I mentioned this earlier, but it's worth a closer look. One of the most common barriers I see around women and exercise is the belief that only certain kinds really count. This can really limit progress towards an active lifestyle, as it means that you are devaluing what is already working well, and telling yourself a story about how you're not truly an active person.

Let's lay this troublesome myth to rest once and for all. For something to count, it simply needs to involve moving your body. More and more studies are finding that the amount of time we spend sedentary is harmful to health, independent of how much we exercise, which means that we *all* need to be moving more, no matter the speed.

In 2011, the *American Journal of Preventative Medicine* published a systematic review[15] (ie the gold standard in research terms) of 48 separate studies examining the impact of sedentary behaviour on health, with 'sedentary time' classed as including general sitting, screen time (including TV time) and other sedentary behaviours. A consistent relationship was found between sedentary time and mortality / weight gain, and while this is perhaps not very surprising in and of itself, the review also went on to conclude that:

> *'There is a growing body of evidence that sedentary behaviours may be a distinct risk factor, independent of physical activity, for multiple adverse health outcomes in adults.'*

What this means in basic terms is that moving your body matters. The more you move your body to do anything other than just sitting, the more you reduce your risk of health problems.

So, all activity counts!

Cardio and strength fitness

In terms of physical activity for fitness, there are two main types: cardio fitness for the heart and lungs, and strength fitness for the muscles and bones.

Public Health England recommends 150 minutes of moderate cardio-type exercise every week. This is essentially any type of exercise that gets you slightly out of breath, so it's not about speed or ability, it's about effort. You can count walking, carrying shopping bags, walking upstairs and gardening IF they get you out of breath. As you get fitter, it gets harder to get out of breath, so you will naturally be able to do more.

The second type of fitness is strength. The current recommendations are to include some kind of strength-building twice a week, and this does become more important for women as we pass the mid-life point. This is where weight-bearing exercises such as yoga can be great to try, and you may even be tempted into a gym for some expert instruction. Equally, there's a wide range of bodyweight exercises freely available on YouTube. Just scroll through to find a suitable beginner's level to start with.

So, my message to you is that you're not to beat yourself up if you need to go on a family walk instead of hitting the gym. Try some faster-paced walking, and if you're with young kids then chase them around. They'll love it, and you'll probably get a better workout than you would have done in the gym anyway.

Improving your fitness isn't about ability, it's about attitude. It's time to take back the wonderful gift that our bodies provide for us, an ability to move and nurture our wellbeing through physical activity. Our bodies are designed for it, and they love it. A body tired from physical activity will sleep better, eat better, recover, regenerate and grow stronger. It's what it's programmed to do. In fact, movement, along with sleep and nourishing food, is a way of recharging your body, in much the same way that plugging in your phone charges the battery, with the key difference being that we usually need to unplug and get out in order to recharge!

A body can't tell the difference between pulling weights in the gym or pulling weeds in the garden, just as it doesn't differentiate between running around the park or running to the shops. All of that judgement and uncertainty comes from our minds.

We can still aspire to the luxury holidays and the spa retreat days, but with the knowledge that these experiences are far more rejuvenating for generally active bodies. The key is to weave more movement into how we live our everyday lives, rather than just seeing it as another chore, or an aspiration for when we have more time and money.

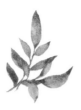

Ready to move?

Our bodies really were born to move, and the more physical activity we can blend into life the better we will feel. Just like how we can't leave a car sitting idle for months at a time, and then still expect everything to work properly when we decide to go for a drive, we've got to keep our bodies moving.

Let's remind ourselves why modern life is so bad for our bodies:

- It's only in the past 200 years that humans have moved as little as we do now. Our bodies are built to conserve energy, and to move far more than many of us do

- 'Fitness' has become a category separate from 'life,' made off-putting by insecurities about doing it wrong or it being too much hard work. In truth, our lives need more movement in them, and that can look like gardening, walking, playing with the children, walking the dog, dancing or anything else that gets us moving

- Current recommendations are for 150 minutes (2.5 hours) of moderate cardio activity and two sessions of strength-building activity each week. This doesn't have to be as daunting as it sounds, especially once you consider ways of bringing 'fitness' back in line with 'living.'

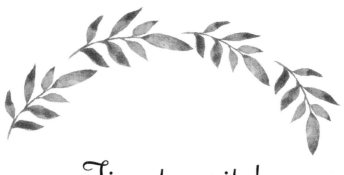

Time to write!

Before you leave this chapter, have a go at the activity below, and see what movement you can reclaim into your life this week:

1. First, let's check-in. Do you feel entitled to move?

   _____

2. Thinking back over the past week, write down every kind of physical activity you did (anything that involved moving your body, either indoors or outside).

   _____

   _____

   _____

   _____

   _____

3. Decide whether you think any of these activities were cardio (getting out of breath) or strength-based (lifting or moving weight).

4. Circle the cardio, and draw boxes around the strength-based.

5. What do you notice about your current movement habits? Are you doing more or less than you thought? Do you have any ideas about how to incorporate more if you'd like to?

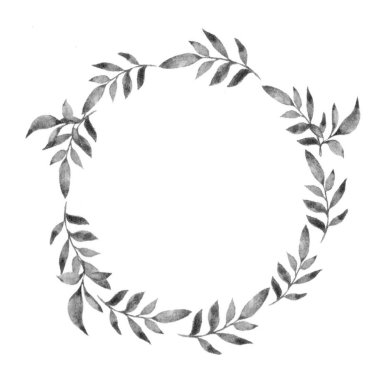

CHAPTER FIVE

You Are Good Enough Already

We're now going to look at how we might be putting up barriers to getting started with exercise and movement. I'm going to explode some common myths, while reminding you that it is your right to move, and to enjoy moving, on your own terms. There are no prizes for doing fitness the 'right' way.

You may not know it yet, but you are good enough already; for exercise, for fitness and for whatever else you want to do. The first thing you need to move is... your mind.

Plan to jump the first hurdle

When we think about a new health drive, we usually focus on what we will do once we are actively pursuing our goals. We make broad, sweeping statements like, 'I'm never going to drink again,' 'I'm cutting out sugar,' or 'I'm going to run a marathon.'

This sets us up to fail, as we ignore the 'getting started' phase of our new lifestyle, and the enormous change in thinking that it requires. Our brains are programmed to resist change, so unless there is a huge emotional motivation driving us, we often fall at the first hurdle.

Failing doesn't mean we are bad at giving up alcohol, eating healthy food or sticking to an exercise routine, but rather that we are bad at planning for change, probably because we have never learned how. Luckily, planning for change is something we can learn to do at any age.

When our brains are busy trying to 'protect' us from change, they become extremely adept at justifying why the plan shouldn't be executed. See if any of the following sound familiar to you:

I can't start a fitness routine because...

- I'm too old
- I'm too big
- I'm too heavy
- I'm too ill
- I'm too unfit
- I'm 'not good' at exercise
- I'm not coordinated enough
- I've not got time

If none of those look familiar, how about:

I'll start exercising when I've...

- Lost some weight
- Recovered from my injury
- Got more time
- Finished that work project
- Got through the holiday season
- [insert any other plausible-sounding excuse here]

When our subconscious is protecting us from change, it can be deceptive. We will believe the reasons we give ourselves, but it's important to remember that this doesn't make us bad, gullible or lazy. It's just part of being human.

Fortunately, there are ways to overcome our natural resistance to change. In fact, this is the foundation of the work I do with my own clients. When our brains instinctively give us reasons why not, we need to proactively remind ourselves of the reasons why; the things in life that really matter to us, and the ways in which the change will help make them better. For some people, getting active is about managing symptoms or improving recovery from an illness, while for others it's about enjoying a healthy later life, or even just being able to chase the kids around the park.

The greatest motivators are those that are personal to us and our own circumstances. When we tap into what really drives us on an emotional level, it propels us forwards with far greater power than before.

Remember back in Chapter One, when I invited you to look at what was most important to you, and to write it down? It's those deep-lying motivations that we're talking about now. They're what you need to come back to every time the hurdles seem too high.

The Truth About Exercise

The truth is that you are always good enough to begin a fitness plan, and you don't have to wait for anything before starting. How do I know this? Because 'exercise' is a very broad term, and too vague to have a real meaning. For example, five minutes walking is exercise. Are you too old, too big or too ill to walk for five minutes? Even if you answer yes to that, are you too old, too big, or too ill to do two minutes of seated chair exercises? Most people reading this can easily do both of these, and whether you're in the category of starting at two minutes or five, a slow start is still better than staying still.

So, it's time to think more broadly. Yes, your injury may be preventing you from going running, but could you do yoga while you heal? Yes, you may not be coordinated enough to follow a Zumba routine, but guess what? The important thing isn't getting the steps right, it's raising your heart rate, and that doesn't require any coordination whatsoever (in fact, it's often more fun without it).

Remember what was said in the last chapter? Our bodies are born to move. Whatever their shape or size, and even with disabilities, chronic conditions and age as limiting factors, they are designed for movement, and so, with suitable adaptation where needed, there is always something we can do. The first step is in the mind; in choosing to move.

Recognise resistance for what it is

Often, our reasons for not exercising are merely a disguise for a deeper emotion: shame. Shame is not a word we often use in our daily language, even though it's a feeling that is commonplace. You may be more familiar with feelings of embarrassment, which the *Oxford English Dictionary* defines as, 'shy, uncomfortable or ashamed,' but why should we feel embarrassment and shame about moving our bodies? Where do these feelings come from?

We live in a world where being old, unfit, ill or fat isn't considered 'cool,' like, at all! What's more, we are constantly bombarded with reminders of this fact through advertising, films and social media, which can turn going out to get fit in public into something of a shame-fest, as not only do we feel like we are on show, but the fact we are exercising is like tacitly admitting that we need to change in order to meet these prevailing standards. Also, many of the clothes that we think we should be wearing in order to do exercise 'properly' will often add to these feelings of embarrassment.

As discussed in Chapter Three, we are forever being sold the idea that it is desirable to be slim and healthy while putting in minimal effort, and as a result, being large and unhealthy, and putting real effort into exercise – especially if we're not doing it in a high-status way, eg with an expensive personal trainer – is perceived as being a potential source of embarrassment. Thus, it becomes a tough topic to talk about; much easier to say that we'll exercise when we've lost some weight, or that we're too old, or we'll do it when our injury heals. These excuses may bring a sense of comfort in the short-term, but they won't benefit our long-term health and wellbeing.

Feelings of embarrassment aren't anything to fear, nor is it a good idea to compound their impact by blaming yourself for having them. There are big social and cultural forces at play that are promoting shame and embarrassment for women and their bodies, and while most people know me as a fairly relaxed person, this is an issue that really makes me angry. You have every right to do as you please with your body, and to enjoy life to the full. No one else's judgement should ever get in the way of this.

If you're able to recognise how embarrassment is getting in the way of your ability to enjoy being active, you must also recognise that this is not your fault. You are entitled to a healthy, active life, and anyone with a negative opinion on that can keep their unhelpful thoughts to themselves!

Honestly, though, in my experience, the population is 98% super supportive of anyone taking action to improve their health. Let's not let the other 2% bring us down.

Let's bust some myths

When our brains send us these vague 'excuses' about why we are not good enough or ready enough to try ANY activity, you can be pretty sure that your subconscious brain is trying to 'help' you resist the change and avoid any possible negative feelings or consequences.

Long-held, deep-seated beliefs are hard to shift, and may require some dedicated work, perhaps even with an exercise psychology coach, but to get you started, first remember that this feeling of shame thinks it's on your side; it is trying to help. The only problem is, it's not helping at all, and is telling some twisted tales to boot, which is why recognising shame for what it is represents a powerful first step.

Now, let's take a look at how it shows up in three common scenarios...

I'm too heavy / too big

Many women tell me that while they would love to exercise more, they are too heavy or too big to start. I also hear women speak about losing weight before they start to exercise.

While I understand the theory behind this approach (lose weight > feel better > start exercising), I think the logic is back to front. As we know, losing weight is often about introducing restrictions to our diet, but in reality, asking someone to avoid alcohol, chocolate and cake is a bit like telling them not to think about a pink elephant. So, if change is already difficult (which it is), we are then adding even further stress by taking the 'Don't do this!' approach. To me, this makes weight loss a difficult path of double resistance, and yes, it is possible to lose weight, but sadly, the resistance often builds to a point where the hard work is then rapidly undone.

To add insult to injury, a failed weight-loss plan is often followed by low self-esteem, due to the person's self-perception of having failed, and low self-esteem is a tough place to maintain a healthy lifestyle from.

But what if we turned this approach on its head?

I advise weight-loss-focussed clients to put their Active Wellbeing first. Why? Because adding activity is a positive focus on adding something in, not taking something away. Increased physical activity can have a rapid positive impact on mental wellbeing, and the subsequent improvement in self-esteem and energy levels gives my clients the boost they need in order to tackle better nutrition if they so wish.

Back in 2006, a review in the journal *Psychology & Health* looked at 121 different studies examining the impact of exercise on body image, and concluded that participation in physical activity is associated with improved body image.[16] This means that my clients are far less likely to choose extreme diets due to the fact that they feel more comfortable in their own skin, paving the way for a more balanced and sustainable approach.

Of course, it's also possible to get active and healthy without weight loss being a factor at all. A stronger body can do more, and cardio exercises strengthen the heart and lungs whatever your size. Add in the mental wellbeing benefits of exercise, and it becomes clear that weight loss is really just a dot on the landscape of getting fitter, as opposed to the main feature that the media and advertising would have us believe. By maintaining a focus on fit instead of fat, we can begin to build our health in a more positive way.

It's fine to acknowledge that there are practical considerations to make when choosing a suitable physical activity, but as we've already established, there are many, many different types to pick from. It's just a case of taking the time to find the right one for you.

I'm too old

We often allow ourselves to believe that exercise is a young person's game. We go through all of that PE at school, and then breathe a sigh of relief when we reach early adulthood, and no one is making us run around a field in our knickers anymore (if you're a post-1990 baby, you were most likely spared being required to do PE in 'gym knickers').

Naturally, as young adults we were invincible, and way too cool for exercise, not least because we were able to stay quite healthy without it, so why bother? However, as we move into our thirties, forties and beyond, we begin to feel less comfortable in our bodies, which could manifest as unexpected weight gain, getting tired more quickly or noticing aches and pains.

These feelings may lead us to believe that our bodies aren't fit for exercise, and so, exhausted from pushing ourselves too hard at aerobics classes and blasting our abs, we opt to decline into old age gracefully. Leave 'shaking your booty' to a younger generation, right?

Wrong.

What I have just described is the typical life journey through exercise for many women. It's a very limited view of what exercise is for and how it works, and yet it shapes the decisions we make about what's the best way to look after ourselves. Having 'been around the block' and 'seen it all before,' we think we've got the fitness and exercise industry figured out, but we forget that many of our experiences of fitness – and this is certainly true of any that took place more than 10 years ago – are based on completely outdated practices and a poor understanding of what actually helps people, especially women, stay active.

These days, there is an extraordinary range of ways to stay active, with more options than ever for the older generations, each adapted to whatever your starting point may be. If you've 'tried' exercise and didn't enjoy it, you simply haven't yet found the right type of activity for you. There is something out there for everyone, whatever their age. You are NEVER too old.

I'm not good at exercise

Exercise isn't a subject that you can pass or fail. If you believe that it is, you can probably blame this on your school PE classes. In sport, there are competitions with winners and losers, but Active Wellbeing isn't a sport. It's solely about improving our physical and mental health.

Going back to the school analogy, being physically active is less like a Maths test and more like an Art lesson; it's not about getting it right or wrong. The joy comes from the doing; from having a go. Yes, you'll probably get better with more practice, but whether your final result is 'good' or not is entirely subjective. Don't become your own harshest critic, as this will take all the fun out of it. When you enjoy what you are doing, you naturally want to do more, and it's the same with fitness and exercise. You can gain pride, self-esteem and confidence from every fitness activity, just as you can from any art lesson. More often than not, the level of 'success' you achieve comes down to whether you are trying to judge the result or simply enjoy the process. I know which one I prefer.

In the UK, the Department of Health recommends that all adults perform 150 minutes of moderate exercise every week[17] (ie 30 minutes a day for five days), and they never add the disclaimer, 'but only if you do it *properly*.'

You need to raise your heart rate and get slightly out of breath, that's it. Coordination, looking good and jogging as far as your friend said she did on Facebook are all completely irrelevant in the pursuit of building fitness.

A healthier and more empowering attitude

I think it's time that we all start changing the way we think about exercise. By working with ourselves at the level we're at now, and not immediately comparing our progress to some far-off ideal, we are much more likely to take encouragement from initial small steps.

Instead of looking at exercise activities and deciding if we can do them, we can look at ourselves and decide which activities fit – not just our level of fitness and ability, but also our lifestyle. Whether we do paid work, have a family, care for elderly relatives or have a dog to walk, we all have factors to consider when planning how and when we're going to exercise. Then, we have our Active Wellbeing goals to consider. Some people want to run a marathon, while others just want to be able to climb the stairs without getting out of breath. Choosing a fitness routine that suits our starting point and OUR goal (not some else's) will make us feel much more motivated.

Lack of time is another major factor, and one we've explored in more detail earlier in the book. All I will say here is decide how much time you have, and then choose the activity to fit, not the other way around. If you worry that you're not doing much exercise, start writing down all the physical activity you do and compare it to the 150-minute government recommendation. If you can increase your activity level by 10 minutes each week, you'll get there in only 15 weeks, even if you begin at zero!

For further support with starting an active lifestyle, check out the resources available at fitbee.co.uk/thelittlebook

The inner critic

I can't finish a chapter about getting started without mentioning the inner critic (also known as negative self-talk), a concept that most women have become all too familiar with in the past 10 years or so. It's nothing new, it's just that we've only now found a label for it, and finally started admitting to one another that this is what we do.

The inner critic is the voice in our minds that tells us what we can't do, what we're no good at and why we're generally worthless. If your best friend spoke to you in that way, you could be sure that she wouldn't be your best friend for much longer, so why do we do it to ourselves?

Once again, it's important to recognise that this is not a failing, but rather a natural mechanism in our brain that seeks to prevent us from trying anything too crazy. We are wired for negativity because our biological evolution hasn't been able to keep up with the rapid changes in our social habits, which is another way of saying that our brains still think that we're going to be eaten by a predator if we set foot outside our caves.

When we treat our inner critic as we would a worried, well-intentioned child, she can be reassured just long enough to demonstrate that she's mistaken in her fears. If we try to argue back, shout down or shut-off this fearful child, we are likely to be faced with a blast of resentment and potentially a torrent of abuse.

Recognise your own inner critic, noticing how she affects your mood and decisions, and how you interact with her. I've already mentioned shame earlier in the book, and this is one of her biggest fears (check out Brené Brown's fabulous research in this area, starting with her *Ted Talk*). Your inner critic will gladly tell you that you're a rubbish swimmer because she worries, *What if someone looks at me?* and the key here is to respond as any responsible adult would to a child: 'I know you're worried, but it's going to be ok. Let's just try – it will be worth it.'

It may also be worth mentioning here the gender gap that exists when it comes to confidence and the inner critic. After all, if it's such a natural process, why do men seem less afflicted? Well, men have exactly the same preservation mechanisms, and they can struggle with change just as much as women, but their fearful child plays out a different storyline shaped by the culture we live in.

A man's fears are driven much more by not wanting to be seen as weak or cowardly, which, when translated into the fitness world, usually means that he's more likely to push himself in a sports environment (or a professional environment, for that matter) because that's the 'strong and brave' thing to do. Ask him to sit in a small group sharing his feelings, however, and you can be sure that he'll soon be talking himself out of it like crazy.

A note on gratitude

To close this chapter off, I'd like to leave you with one final magic potion for quieting negative self-talk, accepting yourself as good enough and beginning your fitness journey:

Gratitude.

Spend some time noticing the things about your body that you are grateful for, and strive to appreciate what it is capable of. Your body is AMAZING! Look at what it's been through and what it's survived, and yet it's still here, turning up every morning and saying, 'Let's have another go, then!'

Practice expressing gratitude for your body, recognising what it does and what it CAN do. Appreciate your body; I mean REALLY appreciate it. How amazing is it that you have a heart beating, lungs breathing, a sense of touch, a nervous system connecting everything together, and a mind that holds consciousness and awareness of yourself and the world around you? Whatever your external circumstances, you are an extraordinary creation with extraordinary powers. Cherish what you have and nurture it.

Reflect on the words of the yoga teacher Vanda Scaravelli:

> *'If you are kind to your body, it will*
> *respond in an incredible way.'*

If right now your body can only allow you a five-minute walk, appreciate it as you gradually build up to 10 minutes. Do this every day, and remember to always enjoy what you already have.

Don't wait for that imaginary future. Live it here and now.

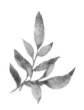

Ready to know that you're good enough already?

If you take only one thing from this chapter, let it be this: you don't need to wait for anything to start moving your body. You can make the choice to get more active right now, even if it's as simple as putting this book down and going for a 10-minute walk, or standing up and spinning your arms in circles. You are good enough already, and your body and mind love you for it.

Love them back.

Time to write!

1. Make a list of three reasons why you haven't felt ready to get active before now.

2. Looking at each reason in turn, give three reasons why this doesn't have to stop you making a start.

CHAPTER SIX

Small Steps Are Bigger Than You Think

We have just explored how you are good enough already, and why you have nothing to prove to anyone before deciding to move more and feel better, but understanding these truths may not make exercise seem like less of a daunting task right away, so it's important to stress again that small steps matter.

As women, we are often self-critical when it comes to assessing our progress, despite being great cheerleaders for everyone else, and this invariably results in us downplaying our own achievements, sometimes without even realising that we are doing it.

For example, I have a friend who, after many months of working on improving her health and fitness, finally achieved her goal of running a 5k for the first time ever. I was so excited and pleased for her, and I told her as much. Then, she responded to one of my messages by saying, 'It was only a 5k.' Needless to say, I quickly replied to make sure that she accepted full credit for her accomplishment.

A woman always needs to be on guard against minimising her own success, as we tend to rob ourselves of the right to celebrate and be proud of the efforts we are making. Every time you take a step forwards, it counts as a win, because remember, we are trying to build an active lifestyle for life. It is not a race; not against ourselves or anyone else.

We're now going to look at actions we can take to move us closer towards our fitness and movement goals, and how these can be approached in ways that make us feel good in the process.

How to prepare for the first step

What's really interesting is how many of us expect change to happen successfully without a plan. How do you feel about change? Some people relish it, others resist at all costs, and most of us fall somewhere in between. For example, how many times have you heard a friend say they'll start a new exercise regime 'on Monday,' or as a New Year's resolution, and then what happens? They might stick to it for a few days or weeks, but they'll most likely fall off the wagon pretty quickly.

Here's the mistake: we wait for the magic date we've set ourselves, and then we just press go.

We wouldn't plan for a holiday this way, would we? Imagine if we decided that we're going on holiday 1st August, and then did nothing about it. We just waited for the date to roll around, woke up and thought, *Right, first day of the holiday*; nothing packed, no idea where to go, nothing booked, not much fuel in the car, half of our best clothes still in the wash, etc.

Do you think our first day on holiday would be a good one? I don't!

Three days later, we're sat in our second-rate hotel (everywhere was booked up), unable to go outside because we only brought warm-weather clothes and it's pouring down, eating supermarket sandwiches because there are no restaurants nearby. We'd be a bit miffed, wouldn't we? What a rubbish holiday!

Would we recognise that our poor planning was at least partly to blame? We probably would, yes, so why don't we recognise how poor planning jeopardises our chances of success when it comes to lifestyle changes?

In Exercise Psychology, we often talk about 'the intention-behaviour gap,' which is the gap between the intention, eg 'I want to be fit and healthy,' and the behaviour, eg 'I regularly exercise to help myself stay fit and healthy.' There has been a lot of research into the intention-behaviour gap[18,19] and how we can overcome it, with consideration of interesting factors such as action planning, coping planning and action control. In layman's terms, the key component is quite obviously planning.

Planning is also a component of something called the 'contemplation' stage of behaviour change,[20] ie the time in which we think about the changes we want to make, where we literally contemplate what it is that we are going to do (for example, I spent a year thinking about writing a book before deciding to do something about it). We can spend years in the contemplation stage, which is why we need a plan of action to help us move forward and bridge the intention–behaviour gap.

The good news is, if you've racked up a few false starts while trying to implement your changes, you can now reframe these failures as research, as we use our experiences to anticipate problems before they happen, and plan ways to overcome them.

The question is, what does a successful plan look like? Some useful areas of planning to consider are:

- How to stay connected to your motivation
- Identifying the types of physical activity that you enjoy
- Anticipating problems and creating contingencies
- Identifying supportive communities for your new lifestyle

This kind of planning is so critical to the prospects of eventual success, I make it the foundation block for all clients starting one of my programmes.

For example, meet Susan. A 42-year-old mum of two, who works part-time. She would love to get fitter, so she came to me for help, and together we looked at why 'getting fitter' had found its way onto her agenda. During the course of our conversation, she realised that it was mostly about not wanting to feel like life was passing her by, as well as wanting to have more energy in all aspects of her life. This was an important realisation, because it helped her to choose which sort of movement to try. We looked at all the types of exercise she'd enjoyed in the past, while pinpointing the periods where she'd felt most alive.

Susan had danced a lot as a girl, and then joined a gym in her twenties, and since she remembered dancing much more fondly than she did her gym membership, she decided that she would start with dance-focussed fitness. With that established, we set two goals: to join a weekly dance class, and to dance to her favourite songs with her toddler in the kitchen every day. We then looked at what potential barriers could have got in her way; one being embarrassment about joining a dance class, as she feared that she'd be the oldest or most unfit attendee.

A solution was found when she joined my Facebook group – a place for women who are happy to say that they're not your picture-perfect gym bunnies! – and asked for recommendations and inspiration. She then found a class not far from where she lived and signed up, and with both me and the group to report back to, she felt supported in her efforts, as she became a shining example of how creating a plan that fits with motivations and lifestyle can, with the necessary support, lead to positive action.

How much exercise is enough?

Now that we've covered the importance of setting ourselves up for success by making a plan, it's time to establish what we are aiming for. This is another area where we can stop ourselves before we've even started if we think we're not capable of doing 'enough,' which is why a key feature of any active lifestyle plan is the amount of exercise we choose to do, albeit keeping in mind that we do not need to tie ourselves in knots with targets.

If we refer again to UK government guidelines, the current recommendation is that all adults do at least 150 minutes of 'moderate' (ie getting slightly out of breath) activity per week. However, it's important to stress that exercise has a 'dose-response' relationship, in that the benefit (response) grows in relation to the amount and intensity of the exercise (the dose). This means that even a few minutes of exercise carries its own (smaller) benefits, and that the amount of benefit increases with the amount of time put in. So, while 150 minutes is great, 60 is still good, and 10 is better than nothing.

Think of it like eating vegetables. We know that we should be aiming for five a day, but if we don't manage that, it's still better to have eaten three portions than none at all (by this logic, trying for seven would give even better results again). Even if you only manage a single carrot, it's still a small step in the right direction, and there's nothing wrong with starting small and building from there.

The same principle applies to housework, learning a new language or gardening. When we look at a task in its totality, it can seem too big; overwhelming, even. This can put us off making a start, but when we concentrate on tidying one room at a time, doing one 20-minute lesson at a time or a quick 10 minutes' weeding, we soon we find ourselves making progress.

However long you choose to spend on exercise, it needs to work for you. Moving your body is about experiencing joy in what you do; if you turn it into a box-ticking exercise, you run the risk of it becoming a chore, and you'll stress over fitting it into your routine. Far better to look for existing opportunities to integrate it into your lifestyle, and to be flexible around the ups and downs of life.

For example, if you have a young baby, you may find it difficult to get to the gym four evenings a week, but that doesn't necessarily mean that you can't do a brisk 30-minute walk with your baby in a pushchair or a sling several times a week, which would be beneficial for both you and your baby.

A little flexibility in our thinking can go a long way.

Set a sustainable pace

As a former long-distance runner, I know all about the importance of pace setting. If you start a race by blasting off too quickly in a burst of enthusiasm, you will inevitably pay for it later on, either by having to stop or struggling to drag your aching body over the finish line. The goal of a long-distance runner is to begin at a comfortable speed, ideally one that feels too easy, and then gradually increase the pace to a level that can be maintained over the full distance.

The same approach should be taken with any lifestyle change. You need to pace yourself!

This begins with two important elements: setting achievable goals, and not looking too far ahead. Let's look at each of these in turn.

What are achievable goals? Remember, you can't control outcomes because you can't control the external factors that sometimes get in the way – after all, life happens – but what you can control are your own actions and behaviours. So, rather than setting speed or distance goals, I recommend 'process goals.' These are the steps that you can definitely take, eg 'I will exercise three times a week,' or 'I will phone up to get details about that fitness class.'

Start from wherever you happen to be. If you currently find a 30-minute walk difficult, begin with a regular 20 minutes instead. Your goal could initially be a 20-minute walk three times a week, and then, after a few weeks, you could increase it to four times, or making one of the walks longer, and so on and so forth.

Although 150 minutes a week is a helpful guideline, it is less important than noticing how your own body feels. You may feel great doing 60 minutes of exercise a week, or you could end up pushing all the way to 200. Everyone is different, and our capacity for physical activity varies with life circumstances, so be kind to yourself. Do what you can, listen to your body and be proud of everything that feels good.

Some people get really excited and motivated by setting themselves big goals for six or 12 months into the future, like signing up for a marathon. If this is you, use it to your advantage; let the big goal motivate you rather than daunt you, but don't neglect those initial small steps. Every big goal needs to be broken down into bite-size pieces, letting you know what you need to do each day in order to move that little bit closer to where you want to be.

There is power in focussing on the present moment. You can't control the future, but you can control the decisions you make now, and the actions that you take today. The future is always being created in the present moment. The time for action is now.

Comparison is the thief of joy

So far, we've talked a lot about keeping focussed on your own goals, your own body and your own likes and dislikes, but how do we actually do this in a society designed to have us make comparisons all the time? It bears repeating that making us feel worse about our bodies is a multi-million-dollar industry.

We often associate fitness with competition. This could be a result of competitive sport being held up as an elite pursuit, schools assessing PE a certain way in the past or the imaged-focussed fitness influencers that dominate social media and lifestyle TV programming. However, a competitive mindset is usually counter-productive when it comes to personal fitness, even if we're only competing with ourselves.

Competition is all about comparison – winners and losers, successes and failures. Now, if your goal is to win, and nothing else matters, that's fine, but if your goal is to live a healthy, active lifestyle and improve your sense of wellbeing along the way, terms like 'loser' and 'failure' are not going to be helpful. At the end of the day, we can't be winners *all* the time!

Besides, why does it matter if your friend goes to the gym twice a week and you do yoga at home? Does that make your fitness levels any poorer? Does it invalidate the great wellbeing benefits that you're gaining? No, absolutely not! In fact, turn the tables, and I'm willing to bet that your friend is wondering if she should do more yoga like you. We all have self-doubt, and we all make comparisons. Let's just be aware of this and catch ourselves when we're doing it, so that we can laugh it off as nothing to worry about.

The use of social comparisons as a means of motivating us to engage in physical activity is now common practice, thanks largely to health and fitness apps. It's thought that by sharing and comparing progress with peers, we feel more motivated to keep going, but while this can be an effective tool for many, it doesn't work for everyone, and it doesn't work all of the time either. Research into Social Comparison Theory has shown that we are risking our self-esteem by regularly comparing ourselves to those who we feel are doing better, and that our responses to it depend on our present state of mind.[21] So, making comparisons is helpful when it feels helpful, but what matters most is your own progress in relation to your personal goals. None of us can live anybody else's life; we have to live our own.

Let's look at another example. Maybe you are out walking every day, whereas your friend is sat in the pub. Does that mean you have a perfect lifestyle? No, it just means that this is where you are now, and only you can decide if you want to do more or less. What your friend is doing isn't relevant to that choice. All you need to ask yourself is, how is your walking making you feel? If it's bringing joy, you may want to do even more. If it's making you feel grumpy, you may be better off finding a new activity, or at least mixing things up a bit. One day, your friend may join you instead of going to the pub, but that's her decision.

One area where it can be helpful to make comparisons is in looking at how far you've come, particularly in regard to your self-awareness and mindset. We all become wiser as we go through life, and even though it isn't always easy to observe or quantify, your growing wisdom is still there, ready to be unleashed when you allow it. Sometimes, looking back on the past can cause feelings of frustration, but thinking about what we used to be able to do, or how much easier it all felt, doesn't exactly help our present state of mind. You have to start from where you are today; there is no other option, so use your experience and wisdom to move yourself forwards.

In the quest for greater wellbeing, comparisons with others are of little value. It's great to celebrate milestones and achievements, but these are only fleeting moments, with the opportunity of more great moments yet to come. Success in competition is built on these milestones, but success in life comes from the journey, and how you feel throughout it.

The power of habits

If at one extreme of the exercise spectrum is training for big events, at the other is forming habitual patterns that blend physical activity into everyday life. Habit forming is what unlocks a consistently active lifestyle. It is what happens when the brain sees something being done so often, it begins to figure out a shortcut. It wants to do it without having to think about it.

We also create habits when we feel rewarded for performing an action. This is how 'bad habits' become so established, as they're normally accompanied by an immediate reward in the form of a pleasurable sensation due to triggering a dopamine release in our brains. It's why so many of us are addicted to our phones, and particularly to social media. A 'like' is a little dollop of dopamine telling our brains, 'This is good, let's keep doing it.' As previously mentioned, our brains are pretty bad long-term thinkers, which is why sugar, alcohol and fast food tend to sneak up our lists of habits.

However, like most powers, habits can be used for good, too. Developing a habit that benefits us in the longer term may require a bit more effort initially, but the pay-off comes when the desired behaviour begins to happen without it really being thought about. By this method, we can create and embed habits that make an active lifestyle feel easy and natural.[22]

Building positive habits

We train our brains constantly via the choices we make. When we repeatedly make a choice that seems rewarding, like having a tasty chocolate biscuit with our morning coffee, our brain believes that it's on to a good thing, and so a habit is quickly formed.

By understanding how the brain works, we can use this habit-forming tendency to our advantage. When we set out to make a lifestyle change, we know that we will have to make a conscious decision to do something that doesn't come naturally. Cavemen were never expected to go run around in the rain purely for the sake of getting some exercise; their motivation for being active was the pursuit of food and shelter. That's no longer the case for us, though.

The key is to deliberately link new activities to immediate positive rewards, thus making them more appealing. Celebrating our running attempt with friends on Facebook will give us a positive buzz, feeling energised for the rest of the day helps justify getting up early for the gym, and 10 minutes' peace from the kids makes that walk around the block seem all the more attractive. The point is, we choose our own rewards when we choose what to focus on, and if we do this often enough, the brain will begin habit forming, which makes getting out of the door a little easier each time.

Now that you know how habits are created, what can you link your desired habit to in order for it to trigger an immediate reward? For example, a walk outdoors could be followed by a hot drink, 10 minutes of strength exercises may be what gives you permission to watch a favourite TV programme, or maybe you'll just dance around the kitchen to your favourite music, a reward in and of itself.

Another good tactic is linking, or 'piggybacking,' two habits together to really make use of our brain's shortcutting ability. While brushing our teeth, could we be marching on the spot? While loading the dishwasher, could we be bending our knees to do squats? When we put the kettle on, could we also put on our favourite music and dance around the kitchen? We saw earlier in the book that the key to Active Wellbeing is building it into everyday life, and piggybacking is a great way to make that happen.

Habits can be your best friends, as well as tricky enemies, so it's definitely worth setting an intention to cultivate the ones that will enhance your wellbeing in the long-term.

The 1% rule

Another really useful way to gradually build up good habits is by using the 1% rule. Imagine if you made just the smallest change, only a 1% difference, to what you currently do. It doesn't seem much, and it should feel very easy, but by making the tiniest 1% progress each day, you could have made a 30% improvement by the end of one month, and 90% after three.

Let's say you've worked out that you do around half an hour's cardio per week at the moment, usually spent running after the kids, and you want to get up to the recommended 150 minutes. Simply make the time to do an extra 30 seconds of getting out of breath each day. Thirty seconds is realistic for anyone, achievable by jogging on the spot while waiting for your friend to answer the zoom call, or for your other half to put their shoes on. Build up from there, and you'll easily get to your 150 minutes a week before you know it.

Eventually, small steps become giant leaps, and this is a principle that applies to habits, too. A habit is normally something that builds up gradually over time; you didn't binge-watch Netflix the first time you switched on your TV, did you? No, you started watching a few programmes you liked, and then you developed a habit of watching a TV at a certain time, which led to seeking out programmes to watch at this certain time, etc.

Let's do the same thing with our positive habit-building. Would you like to have a daily walk routine? Great! How about you walk to the corner shop once a day? Then, once you've run out of things to buy, make it a walk around the block, followed by a 15-minute walk, and then a 15-minute walk plus walking to the corner shop when you need to buy something again. Small, incremental steps that involve doing the easiest things possible will help build confidence through regularity, which will later form a habit.

Oh, and don't forget that hot drink when you get in from your walk, too!

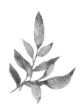

Ready to take small steps?

It's easy to get overwhelmed with the size of the task at hand when it comes to improving our fitness and wellbeing. From the bottom of the mountain, it looks like a long and difficult journey, with the summit never seeming to get closer, which is why we need to focus on the process; on the small steps we take.

Moving is moving, whether we're at the start of a journey or near the end, and what is the end anyway? We don't need to have a goal to get active in three weeks or three months; we can get active today by standing up and walking out of the front door.

Change happens in the now, and every step counts.

Time to write!

1. What negative / unhelpful habits do you have in regard to your Active Wellbeing?

    _____

    _____

    _____

    _____

2. What positive habits would you like to create?

    _____

    _____

    _____

    _____

3. Choose one positive habit, and write down how you could begin to include this in your life. Think about the smallest, most manageable change, and then do it!

_____

_____

_____

_____

_____

_____

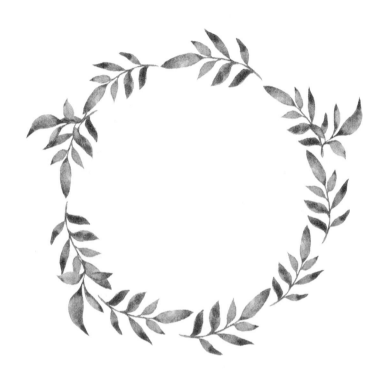

CHAPTER SEVEN

Connection Is Key

When we think about our health and wellbeing, for most of us there are a few themes that come to mind first. Food is normally the big one, with exercise following close behind, and then, increasingly over the past few years, we have become more aware of the importance of mindfulness, stress management and the ever-ubiquitous phrase self-care. However, there remains one element of wellbeing that is frequently overlooked:

Connection.

Actually, maybe I should say that connection *was* overlooked, as due to the COVID pandemic Lockdowns, the world has experienced its biggest ever reminder of how important it is. As we became cut off from our loved ones, the popularity of online connection tools surged; Facebook, Zoom, Google and Microsoft (among others) were falling over themselves in a race to become the online meet-up platform of choice, as suddenly even Nana had a Zoom account!

This showed us something that deep down we already knew, but had perhaps taken for granted; that a sense of connection matters to us humans. Feeling connected contributes to our sense of wellbeing, and feeling disconnected does just the opposite.

In this chapter, I will explore three elements of connection, and how being physically active can play an important role in enhancing all of them. These are connection with self, connection with others and connection with the natural world.

Connection with self

One of the biggest issues I come across with the women I coach through my wellbeing practice is a loss of connection with self. It's a particularly cruel state to be in; it leaves the sufferer feeling lost, joyless and tired, to the point where they think there's something wrong with them. If only they could see what I see; the towers of strength that they are. They would know that it's an extremely common phenomenon among women, and especially mothers, whose lives are so incredibly busy; there's always something to get done. Life commitments can make us lose touch with our own preferences, thoughts, imaginations and desires, until finally we are no longer sure who we are anymore. Throw into the mix society, family and cultural expectations, and it's no surprise that many of us wake up one day wondering who we are and how we got here.

I had this experience myself back in 2014, when I returned to my high-flying management job following the birth of my son two years earlier. I'd been back at work around 12 months, and I was experiencing for the first time the tightrope that all new mums have to walk when they try to mix career and family. I was sent off to the Netherlands for a Women in Leadership programme, and as part of the course we did an exercise on identifying our values; our core values; our personal values; what really makes us tick. It should have been a simple task, but I was astonished to discover that I had no idea what my values were anymore. This was the moment I realised that I had lost connection with myself. I no longer knew who I was or what I wanted.

I had been working so hard to achieve something, and now I didn't even know why. I was lost. It was a big shake-up moment for me, and I know that it happens to millions of other women, too.

How can physical activity help?

There is a solid, tangible nature to physical activity, which makes it a great way to commit to ourselves. Often, self-care habits such as taking baths, meditating and reading can slip when others in the home are making demands on our time, and so committing to some sort of workout, especially one that gets us out of the house, makes it clear that you are taking a slice of time for yourself. This lays the groundwork for self-connection, as you are allowing yourself the space and freedom to be you. It's also harder for the kids to interrupt you when you're out walking than if you're in the bath!

Moving your body forces you to pay closer attention to it, and paying attention is the first step towards reconnection. This time spent in your body, rather than in your head, can free your mind from some of the noisiness of life, and bring you back to you. It's a very similar principle to meditation, but in a more active form.

Of course, some types of physical activity work better than others. For example, swimming, walking and running don't typically require much thinking about the movements involved, leaving you free to focus on how you are feeling, and to listen to the sounds and sensations around you. A vigorous spin class is likely to be less peaceful, but it still brings the sensation of breathing, as well as feelings in the legs and the lungs that will demand your attention, even if you don't focus on them intentionally.

Physical exertion nudges you to notice your body and how it is feeling, which helps you to connect to yourself in a compassionate, positive way. It's an opportunity to cultivate an attitude of thankfulness for what your body can do, and is an extremely uplifting practice for helping you to appreciate what a wonderful creation you are.

Additionally, physical movement also creates a sense of freedom and autonomy, as we saw when we explored the importance of putting your own oxygen mask on first in Chapter Two. Giving yourself permission to do something for yourself, in whatever way you choose to do it, provides a sense of control that could be missing from other parts of your life. It reminds you that you have freedom of choice, and that you can make your own decisions in life.

The sense of freedom gained from being more active can ripple into other areas, too. Take, for example, my friend

Gayle, who tells me that she gets her best blog and business ideas when she is running, which doesn't surprise me. As far back as 1997, the *British Journal of Sports Medicine* was reporting that creative thinking is significantly increased following exercise, citing research carried out using an aerobic dance video. Since then, further studies have confirmed the positive impact of exercise on mood and creativity, especially in relation to jogging, running and even dancing![23]

Gayle was also amazed at the improvement in her strength and stamina over time, achieved simply by sticking with it, which further demonstrates the power of small steps. She believes that through the straightforward process of learning to run, she learned an important lesson about how anything she wanted was within her grasp if she chose to put the time and commitment in. Gayle still considers running to be a business activity (as do I), although she's not had the guts to claim running shoes as a business expense yet!

Connection with others

There is a wonderful relationship between physical activity and connecting with other people. For starters, becoming more physically active creates more opportunities to socially connect to others, and to share a similar interest beyond discussing the weather, but there's more to it than that. Creating a sense of community is also a key motivational component in helping get you started with being active and encouraging you to maintain it long-term.

This is why places like running clubs, walking clubs and cycling clubs are so popular. It is possible to do every one of these activities on your own (indeed, it's part of their appeal for many), but being part of a club (or community) brings with it a social support network to keep you going, as you share your struggles and successes. Even during Lockdowns, many of these clubs have gone online, launching weekly challenges, social quizzes and virtual events to keep their members connected.

Humans are wired to seek out a sense of belonging. It comes from the times where we sought safety in numbers, as we relied on one another in our quest to hunt and gather food, and also for protection against both predators and rival tribes. For these reasons, it was always better to be part of a group, and to this day, the primitive parts of our brains equate belonging with safety.

There is just something naturally appealing about being part of something greater than ourselves, even if we prefer to sit on the edge of the tribe looking in. Finding common ground with members of the group, such as through shared interests and attitudes, adds to this sense of belonging, not least because it makes it less likely that we'll be kicked out.

In the modern world, this explains why we enjoy joining clubs or communities for people with shared interests, even when those interests appear to be solitary pursuits. A community conservation project or local sports event may bring people together only briefly, but it's enough to provide everyone with positive psychological benefits, as they come away feeling like they've had a good day.

It's difficult to overstate the importance of community when it comes to getting started and keeping going with regular exercise. Yes, many people manage without it, but motivation is made easier by adding a sense of community to the mix, in whatever quantity you feel comfortable with. It doesn't have to be an official club, either. You may happen to come across people who want to join you in your new endeavours, and this could eventually lead to genuine friendships that go beyond being just exercise buddies. Family members can also be a great source of support, though I would advise not relying solely on one person alone, as this may cause issues if one of you has to stop for any length of time. For that reason, a network is much more reliable.

If you don't have a ready-made community for your activity of choice, where do you start? Well, for all of its many evils, this is where social media can play a really powerful and positive role. It won't take much searching on Facebook to find a group dedicated to your activity of choice, with a network of likeminded people on hand to chat with you for hours on end. Of course, you are also always welcome to join my Active Wellbeing Community, a place where you can discuss the ideas raised in this book in much greater detail.

Even if Facebook isn't your cup of tea, it can point you towards other websites, local clubs and sporting governing bodies offering a wealth of information. Someone once said to me that there is no longer a problem that can't be solved by asking Google, and while I'm not sure that's completely true, it's certainly a big help when searching for your activity tribe.

Connection with the natural world

Finally, we come to physical activity's third connective power: the ability to help us feel connected to the world we live in. Moving our bodies helps us tap into the sense that there is something bigger than us; something that we are fortunate to be a part of. When we take part in exercise, or any physical activity for that matter, it gives us a chance to get away from our phones, our desks or our family responsibilities for a short time, allowing us an opportunity to spend time in the wider world.

This is especially true for any activity done outdoors, which is something I strongly encourage due to the additional wellbeing benefits. As we covered in Chapter Three, spending time in nature enables us to reconnect with the space around us, and the planet and environment that is our home. I remember back when I was a keen amateur triathlete, I used to take training very seriously, forever monitoring my sports watch and worrying about my heart rate or how fast I was (or wasn't) going. Eventually, though, I realised that I was missing the point, and nowadays, I positively adore soaking up nature as I run or walk. I stop to look at flowers, and I pause to admire the view. It may knock a few seconds off my time, but to me this matters far less than the enjoyment I gain from reconnecting with nature and finding my own headspace before returning home to family life, and the responsibilities that come with it, completely rejuvenated.

In 2020, the *Journal of Environmental Psychology* published a study involving almost 5000 adults, which investigated the relationship between connecting with nature and our general health and wellbeing. It was found that 'visiting' nature more than once a week was positively associated with better health, as well as a heightened sense of caring about the environment. The study concluded that increasing contact with and connection to nature is likely to be a prerequisite for improving both human and planetary health, or to put it more simply, the more time we spend in the natural world, the more likely we are to care for it, and the healthier we will be.[24]

There are some brilliant ways to combine caring for the environment with physical activity, such as conservation volunteering and green gyms. Try using Google to see what's happening in your local area, as you may have some great opportunities right on your doorstep.

Using our own bodies for transport in the form of walking, cycling or running is also good for the planet. When I was a kid, my family didn't own a car until I was seven years old, and I vividly remember walking everywhere or, if we had to go a bit further, occasionally taking the bus. Lots of people did this back then, and although we occasionally got a soaking in the rain, it was far better for both the planet and our health. Plus, getting wet in the rain is another great way to reconnect with nature!

At time of writing, 'Active Transport' is being featured quite heavily in the news, as part of a government policy to encourage people to travel actively for the benefit of themselves and the environment. Whatever else we think of the government in 2020, encouraging people to move their bodies more is definitely a step in the right direction, so let's get behind it and try to become more creative in how we can get from A to B. The school run is a great place to start; you could choose just one day a week initially to walk or cycle to school, and then build yourself up from there. If it's too far (or inconvenient), think about parking the car further from the school gates, so that you're adding in a short walk each day. Once you begin to see the benefits, you could make it a challenge to set off earlier, as you gradually park further and further away.

Being physically active outdoors also carries lots of money- and time-saving benefits. Rather than going to the cinema or for an expensive meal, why not spend time on a long country walk and take a picnic with you? You will save money and get fitter all at once! As for time saving, how long does it take you to drive to the cinema or gym? The outdoors is literally out the back door (and the front!), with no commuting involved, and if there's one thing we've learned from repeated Lockdowns, it's that there is a wonderful world on our doorstep when we choose to take the time to slow down and appreciate it.

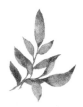

Ready to connect?

Physical activity in any form is a powerful tool for reconnection in our increasingly disconnected world. The mental wellbeing benefits of being able to feel reconnected cannot be understated, whether it's the mother finding herself again, the new retiree finding a new role in life, or the conscientious career woman rediscovering that there is more to life than her 60-hour work week. We all benefit from connection, and physical activity provides us with opportunities to reconnect with life whenever we need it.

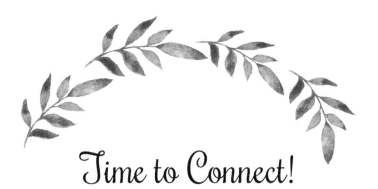

Time to Connect!

I'd like you to commit to doing this mindful movement exercise sometime in the next week, so get your diary out now and pencil it in. Even if the weather's freezing, I encourage you to try it for just a couple of minutes!

Taking the time to notice how you feel before and afterwards...

- Find an open grassy space where you will be left undisturbed. A back garden is perfect, but a quiet park will do just fine.

- After checking for sharp objects on the ground, remove your shoes and socks.

- Close your eyes and gently step forward, feeling the grass beneath your toes and hearing the sounds around you.

- Continue walking for as long as you feel comfortable.

- 10–20 minutes is great, and yes, you can peek to check that you won't crash into things.

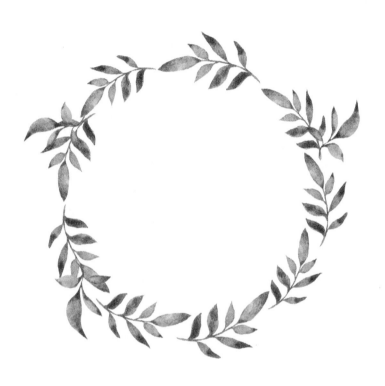

CHAPTER EIGHT

It's About the Journey, Not the Destination

I hope that by this stage of the book, you have come to better understand my views on physical activity and how it shapes our health and wellbeing. This is not about becoming an elite athlete or a fitness fanatic; it's about blending regular exercise and movement into your life in order to make it better for you, for those around you and for the world we live in.

When you move more, you feel better; you have more energy, you want to look after yourself properly, and there is a ripple effect across the rest of your life. It's OK to have phases where things slow down or even stop. In fact, it's not just OK, it's totally normal; all is not lost. We can choose to move forward again at any time, and when we do, the benefits will come.

We're now going to delve deeper into the process of cultivating a nurturing attitude towards your Active Wellbeing. We are so used to seeing fitness, like many other things in life, as a chore, or something that needs to be achieved and ticked off a list, but that misses the point. This is about living well, but how are you going to do that if you're always focussed on when the task at hand will be over? It's about the journey, not the destination.

To goal set or not to goal set?

I do help clients set goals, though I rarely do them for myself anymore. Why is that? Well, there are pros and cons to goal setting, and it is very much a case of right time and place.

Goals are wonderful for a beginner; they provide clear focus and a sense of direction, and when done well, they are broken into small, clear steps that are easily achievable and serve to build confidence. Whenever you feel like a tiny ant at the bottom of a huge mountain, a little goal setting will help get you going, and keep you feeling great about your progress along the way. With small steps, tiny ants climb huge mountains.

So, what's the problem? A goal is all about something we want to achieve in the future, but while that's inspiring for some, it's a distraction for others. Focussing on a future goal can lead us away from the process of doing what needs to be done today. It's like the goal of giving up chocolate or drinking, which could always wait until tomorrow. It's a big goal, and it's scary, but it's happening in the future, so today we can put it off.

Of course, we all know how the future turns out when we keep putting things off, but unfortunately, our brains are programmed to exist in the moment, and so we struggle to conceive long-term risks and instead prefer to focus on what feels good right now. As a result, 'I'm going to run a marathon in six months,' quickly becomes, 'That's ages away. It'll be OK if I have a packet of crisps and watch TV tonight. I'll start training tomorrow.'

One way to counter our ingrained negative habits is to make sure any big goal is broken down into smaller weekly, or even daily, process goals, eg 'I will run three times a week,' or 'I will do 20 minutes exercise every day.' This works much better, though it's not without its own pitfalls. Imagine for a moment that you are a busy working mum, and on your to-do list for the day, you have to get the kids ready, stick some washing on, get to work, pick some shopping up and, oh yes, go for a 20-minute run (I'm giving an easy day as an example).

It's all perfectly planned out, but then you get to work and find out that a colleague is off sick, so you're asked to cover an extra task; there's your lunchtime gone. The school ring, and your son forgot his kit for football after school, can you drop it off? There's your free time after work gone. After a frantic day, you're faced with going for a run OR getting some food in to feed your family, and you have to REALLY be in the zone to hold out and tell the family that it's beans on toast for tea (again).

So, you survived the day, but you missed the run. This actually isn't a big deal – that's life! – but what about your goal? This is where goals can turn the tables on us, as leaving them unmet has us starting to think, *Maybe I'm not cut out for exercise. Maybe I'm too busy to fit it in?*

Do you see how setting a goal that fails can inadvertently push you into a spiral of negative thinking? Yes, goals can be helpful, but they must not be treated as the be all and end all. I prefer journey-focussed goals or intentions.

Journey-focussed goals

One way to avoid the pitfalls of goal setting is to make your goals journey-focussed, or to set an intention.

An intention could be to run at least three times a week, or more if the opportunity presents itself. An intention could be to exercise every day, which means that it matters less if some days get missed. An intention could be to work on strength or stretching on days where you've missed your run. These intentions are more flexible, and yet still provide a clear sense of direction.

Instead of setting a results-based goal such as, 'I will walk the London Marathon,' you set a journey-focussed goal, eg 'I will walk every day.' The journey is what will ultimately determine how you feel about yourself day-to-day, and so it doesn't really matter if the main goal is missed because you will have had plenty of mini wins all through the journey. It's much easier to succeed with journey-focussed goals because they are smaller, and thus more likely to become habitual. You will have something to celebrate each day, which will help to build up your confidence until being active becomes a much more natural and effortless part of how you live your life.

Whether you prefer goals, intentions or something else entirely, the main thing is to know the direction you want to head in, and to take steps towards it. As I explained in Chapter Six, those steps can be small; it's often better if they are. It is the feeling that we are heading in the right direction that creates real joy in life.

The pros and cons of accountability

Accountability is often mentioned by my clients as something that they really need help with if they're to get moving and stay motivated. Accountability is a close relation of goal setting; it's a way to follow-up and see if the goal is being achieved.

Let's pick this apart for a moment. We've set our goal, we've declared for all the world what we want to do, and now we want someone to hold us accountable. The positive side of this is that there is nowhere to hide; another person is now invested in our development, expecting a report and wanting to see some progress.

If you are used to reporting to others, and you enjoy being a people pleaser, this is probably right up your street. You can check-in, say how well you're doing and, if you're lucky, get some praise. This can be a really powerful driver at times where our internal motivation is low, and it certainly helps people get started, but just like with goal setting, there is a downside.

Accountability relies very heavily on external (extrinsic) motivation, meaning that the motivating force comes from outside of you, from the person holding you accountable, so how can you be sure that it's motivating you in the exact way that you need? Obviously, if they're holding you to account for a goal that you set yourself, you're still exercising some control, but our goals can and will change, just as our lives and needs do.

It's actually quite difficult to set-up a system of accountability that is continually responsive to your needs. Why does that matter? Well, because you are doing this for you, and you only! You are the one living your life; you are the one who knows how you feel, and you are the one who knows deep down what you need in order to move forward.

Even the most talented, skilful, and well-intentioned personal trainer or coach will still never be able to truly understand your needs as well as you do, so yes, by all means use accountability if you feel it gives you a boost, but remember that you are the one in the driving seat. This is something that you are doing for yourself, not anyone else.

Note that there is a difference between accountability and community. For example, during the spring / summer 2020 Lockdown, I ran a very successful 'Couch to 5k' group, bringing a group of women together online to support one another on their journey to achieving their running goals. A sense of community helps us to feel inspired and part of something, as there is always someone there to celebrate with when things go well, or to offer support if they take a turn for the worse. Some members of the group might have viewed this as a source of accountability, but the truth is that they were accountable to no one but themselves. There was no expectation and no pressure; I wasn't there with a virtual cattle prod, nudging them off their sofas! It was a place where women could feel a sense of belonging within an atmosphere of acceptance of understanding, with the aim of enabling them to grow in confidence on their own terms.

Your internal (intrinsic) motivation

If external motivation isn't great, what do we have that's better? (I'm glad you asked.) In 2012, a systematic review of 66 empirical studies defined the role of intrinsic motivation in starting and maintaining a physically active lifestyle.[25] Different motivation types exist along a scale, with pure extrinsic motivation at one end and pure intrinsic motivation at the other, with a varying blend of the two in the middle (think the greyscale between black and white).

Every type of motivating force sits somewhere along this scale, whether it's wanting to change our body shape, feel healthier, take part in certain events or climb the stairs without getting out of breath. Each and every desired benefit will be driven by some blend of intrinsic and extrinsic motivation, and as far as long-term maintenance of an active lifestyle goes, the greater the proportion of intrinsic motivation the better.

So, what is intrinsic motivation? Essentially, it's the exact opposite of extrinsic motivation, which is derived from external forces (ie the views, opinions and needs that exist outside of us), whereas intrinsic motivation comes from within. Think of intrinsic motivation as being what gets you to feel motivated even when no one else is looking.

Imagine spending the day being driven solely by extrinsic motivators, and how that would feel. You get out of bed at 7am because that's the time you have to be up for work; you get dressed in a particular uniform that work requires; you catch the bus because your husband wants to use the car; you work a job that your parents think is amazing, but you're not sure you're enjoying it; and you eat a 'slimming' lunch because you think you need a bikini body for your next holiday, since other people will see you on the beach.

Now, compare that to a day spent following intrinsic motivation. You get out of bed at 7am because you're looking forward to the day; you get dressed in a particular uniform, which you love because outfits are now one less thing to worry about, and you think it looks great; you catch the bus because you know it means you'll get to walk more, and you enjoy the fresh air; you work a job that you really enjoy doing because it feels worthwhile; and you eat a light lunch because you know it'll leave you feeling more energised in the afternoon.

Do you see how even with an almost identical set of activities, the difference between intrinsic and extrinsic motivation will feel very different? Of the two examples, which do you think sounds most sustainable?

If you rely on accountability and peer pressure for getting your exercise done, you are probably more extrinsically motivated. If you decide to go for a walk one day and don't even tell anyone about it, you are more likely intrinsically motivated. It's not so much an indication of the type of person you are, but rather how you feel about what you do and why.

We live in an extrinsically motivated society, where employers, schools and even supermarket points schemes offer rewards for the behaviours that they want to see. Intrinsic motivation is harder to spot, but that doesn't mean it isn't there; it's just a matter of tuning into it. We've already explored the ways in which we have become disconnected from our own thoughts and feelings in this busy world, and it's now time to look at how reconnecting and retuning can help us to uncover what it is that really matters to us in life.

One way to reconnect with internal motivation is by listing the benefits of physical activity that matter to you. I challenge you to only choose the benefits that you truly care about, not those that matter to other people, or that you think you 'should' pick. Take a blank piece of paper and write down as many benefits as you can think of (at least 10). This will increase your motivation for exercise. (Sounds too simple? Give it a try and see what happens!)

As you process your thoughts on the benefits, you are reminding yourself that they exist, which in turn brings the reasons for doing them to the forefront of your thinking (just as we did at the very start of this book).

Why I ran an ultramarathon

An ultramarathon is not an obvious choice of activity for a 41-year-old mum with a young child, especially one who was still quite inactive just three months out from the event. I had pushed myself really hard the year before, and I was going through a much-needed recovery break, so I wouldn't have described myself as motivated at all. In fact, if someone had tried to push me into getting more active again, I almost certainly would have resisted, but then I remembered something.

The Haworth Hobble is an ultramarathon spanning 33 miles across the West Yorkshire Moors. My dad had completed it when I was a child, and I decided that I wanted to do it with him when I was around 14 or so. Of course, I was too young to enter then, and unfortunately, by the time I was old enough,

I had stopped running and become much more interested in boys, beer and pizza; the beginning of my decade-long decline into poor health.

I then went through a rollercoaster ride of fitness and non-fitness, focussing mainly on triathlons, and it was during one of my periodic descents that I realised I had an opportunity. I hadn't yet lost all of the previous year's fitness, so maybe, just maybe, at the age of 41, I would still have a base-level high enough to get me to an ultramarathon in only three months. It was a chance to realise a childhood dream, and also to pull off something unexpected, and so I had my deep intrinsic motivation. There was zero external pressure, and it certainly had nothing to do with trying to look good – most people have never even heard of the Haworth Hobble – I really was just doing it for me.

I started training far too late, leaving myself only eight weeks to prepare (do not try this at home!), and it was 2018, the year it kept snowing all through February and March. That was when I did my 12- and 17-mile training runs; my husband and son would drop me off in the middle of nowhere, and I'd try to run / walk / crawl back. I arrived on 'race day' thinking the same thing I always do at these big events: *I have no idea if I'm going to make it or not.*

Long story short: it was tough, but I made it, as the intrinsic motivation of a childhood dream drove me 33 miles through rain, peat and snow. Ten hours later, I finished the race, tired but very content!

If intrinsic motivation can do that for me, it can definitely help you discover a happier, healthier and more active lifestyle. It's just a case of finding how to tap into it, and then connecting with what really matters to you.

Keeping the positive outcomes in focus

Because our brains are so good at scanning for danger and negative consequences (to keep us safe), it is important that we remind ourselves of the positive outcomes we are working towards. Visual reminders are a useful way to do this, so try seeing if any of the following tasks sound appealing to you as a way of creating your own personal motivation booster (when you have chosen one or more, you can then set aside an hour or two for some creative fun):

1. **Create a digital image for your phone or laptop**

   Choose something that represents the driving force behind your goal, and use it as a screensaver or post it around social media. If you don't want to create your own, you can search the internet for phrases or images that capture how you feel.

2. **Motivation-boost your home!**

   Got a catchy image or phrase that will help drive you on? Use it in your home decorating! You can get printed mugs, fridge magnets, key rings, cushion covers... I'm sure you could think of more, or alternatively, go low-tech and use sticky notes. You can choose something that's small and private, or you can plaster it all over your house; it's completely up to you. The main thing is that you create something you will see regularly, and that you will know what it means to you.

3. **Create your own work of art or vision board**

   Photos, images, drawings and paintings can all be really powerful ways of embedding ideas into the brain. It's not just the image you're left with, but also the process of creating it, which will help the messages sink into your subconscious. Try to capture in pictures the future life and feelings you're working towards, and why it's important to you. If you're not feeling artistic, vision boards can also be created by cutting out pictures and phrases from magazines. Alternatively, digital versions can be sourced from websites like Pinterest.

Enjoy the journey

Whatever strategies or tactics you use to make your active lifestyle happen, it's super-important to keep in mind that enjoyment and wellbeing in everyday life is the main goal. Stay mindful of your intentions about how you want to feel; stay aware of the ups and downs, the good days and bad days, remembering that they all have a role to play; they are part of the journey. No matter how many false starts or setbacks you have, you can stay motivated and keep moving forward by focussing on what's truly important to you.

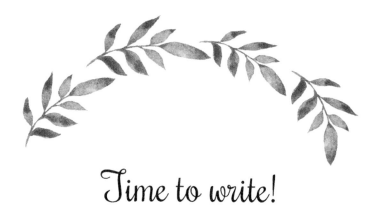

Time to write!

1. As you begin your journey towards a more active lifestyle, consider how you would you like this process to feel (circle all words that apply, and don't hesitate to add more if you have them):

Fun	Challenging	Inspiring
Tough	Hard work	Enjoyable
Rewarding	Happy	Content
Relaxing	Restful	Interesting
Exciting	Fresh	Familiar
Stretching	Comfortable	Community
Freeing	Amazing	Entertaining

2. Using two or three of your answers, complete the following sentence to create a declaration of your intentions for your journey:

I intend that my journey to a more active lifestyle should feel

---

CHAPTER NINE

Mind the Gap

$Good$ intentions are great; they're where everything starts, and hopefully, if you've read this far, you're feeling good about the benefits that Active Wellbeing brings. However, the fact remains that in order to turn intentions into reality, we need to take action.

Bridging the intention-action gap

The intention-action gap is perhaps one of the biggest barriers that stands between where we are now and the active, healthy lifestyle we'd love to have. Fortunately, the Seven Principles of Active Wellbeing shared in this book each form a piece of the bridge that crosses this gap, and you can use them to help get yourself started, and to strengthen your resolve if ever you feel yourself flagging at any time.

Each principle comes with a short complementary activity, to help you understand, strengthen and solidify its message in your mind. Take a look now to see whether or not you've completed them all, and if you haven't, set a date in your diary to do so. Remember, these tasks should only take 20–30 minutes each, so if you are struggling to get started, consider it a step on your journey towards getting moving.

Trust me, it'll be worth it.

Activity Checklist	Chapter	Page	Done
'Where are you now?' check-in	1	24	
Understanding your thought patterns	1	26	
Why do you want to live a more active life?	1	27	
Put on your own oxygen mask first	2	43	
It's about how you feel, not how you look	3	55	
You were born to move	4	68	
You are good enough already	5	86	
Small steps are bigger than you think	6	102	
Connection is key	7	115	
It's about the journey, not the destination	8	129	

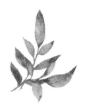

Completed the Tasks? Ready for Action?

Great, you're ready to get moving, so now what? What's the best way to make it happen? You need a plan.

The key elements of a good Active Wellbeing plan are competence, autonomy and relatedness. These are the main components of Self-determination Theory, and they have all been shown to improve motivation to exercise.[5,26]

Here is a breakdown of what the three components mean, and how you can blend them into your planning:

Competence

Perhaps the most straightforward of the three, competence is literally about how capable you feel when performing a particular task. The more confident you are in your abilities, the more likely it is that you will enjoy whatever you're doing, which will increase the likelihood of you feeling motivated to keep going.

So, what does this mean for your Active Wellbeing?

It means that you should start from wherever you happen to be right now, and take small steps. The simplest and easiest activities that you can think of are the best ones to start with; far better to aim for one press-up a day and achieve it than to go for ten and feel like you've failed if you only manage five.

If you want to try something new, find a very patient and friendly trainer or coach to take you through the basics and help you to master them. Another option could be joining a class at a suitable beginner's level (so many people sign up for high-intensity gyms or personal trainers, and then cancel because it seems too hard).

Start on easy mode every time.

Autonomy

I have to say, this is my favourite component, and I'm sure it's popular with many other women, too. Autonomy is about being able to choose for yourself, and this can apply to anything from the activities you do to the times you do them, as well as the goals that you set for yourself.

It's important to make sure that you are in charge of the decisions you make, as it's all too easy to hand over responsibility to someone else, thinking that they'll do the hard work for us. A good example of this is signing up with a PT who can 'Just tell me what to do,' or blindly following the latest social media trend because 'It's what everyone else is doing.'

When we make our own decisions, we are not only much more invested in the outcome, but also far more likely to have chosen something that suits us and our lifestyle. So, how do you blend autonomy into a plan? By creating a plan of your own! That's why I teach my clients how to develop their own plans, rather than writing one out for them.

There are countless free training and exercise plans available on the internet these days, but none of them are tailored to you and your needs. Invest some time in yourself, and come up with something that really works for you.

Relatedness

Relatedness is about your support network; the human interactions that help support the changes you want to make, and the active lifestyle you want to live. This is really wide-ranging, and could include friends, family and connections online (you could probably even count your dog if it's joining in).

As I mentioned in Chapter Seven, we all crave a sense of belonging and connection, and a plan that helps satisfy these needs will ultimately stand a greater chance of being successful. The question is, what practical steps can we take in order to work this into a plan?

First of all, consider how you may be able to interact with others during the activities that you want to do. This could be through joining clubs, classes or groups online, although it's also fine to enjoy solo activities if that's your preference. In this case, is there a way you can share your adventures with people?

Next, think about interactions with family and friends. Do any of them have similar goals to you? Have you asked them? You may be able to support one another through the occasional message or check-in to see how it's going.

Last, but by no means least, where will you get support for the lifestyle changes that you wish to make? Friends and family are great, but if one falls off the wagon, it's good to have backup to prevent a domino effect. You can invest as much or as little into this as you like, with options ranging from free online support groups to personal 1:1 coaching. Personally, I would advise investing as much as you can afford – which perhaps isn't surprising, given my job – but at the end of the day, this is your life we're talking about, and so figuring out how to feel as good as possible while you live it seems a worthwhile investment to me.

Whatever you decide, be sure to look at your plan from the perspective of connecting to others.

Laying out a plan

To be honest, the plan layout isn't especially important as long as it's clear enough for you to follow. There's no perfect blueprint; what's important is that it's meaningful to you.

As an example, here is the layout I currently use with my own clients (Figure 1). This plan has all the information needed, plus a handy tick box for marking when each activity is complete. You can download a PDF of this template for your own use at fitbee.co.uk/thelittlebook

Why you want to be more active			
Weekly Time Target (mins)			
Day	**Time**	**Activity**	**Done**
Mon	12:00 (20mins)	Dancing to the radio	

Figure 1: A Simple Activity Planner

Once you've filled in your plan, that's it. You're ready to go!

Time to plan!

I would now like for you to complete your own Activity Plan. As you decide on goals, bear in mind some of the key teaching aspects from the Seven Principles of Active Wellbeing:

- plan before you act
- do what makes you feel good
- break it down into achievable steps
- focus on the next couple of weeks
- pay attention to what you're doing, not what anyone else is
- build-in relatedness and connection where you can

Assign yourself a quiet 20 minutes, and then write down:

1. The times you have available in the week for being active.
2. The activities you would like to try.
3. A target number of minutes per week for physical activity.
4. Fill in the Activity Planner (download your free copy at fitbee.co.uk/thelittlebook)

And there you have it! An actual plan for your own Active Wellbeing, grounded in the seven important principles shared in this book, but this is just the start.

Now that you've read this book, I hope you, too, can see that there is a more balanced way to approach a healthy, active lifestyle. It's not all about the HIIT workouts, or how fast or far you can run. There are so many different elements of physical activity to enjoy, and I sincerely hope that you take some inspiration and courage from my words as you move forward and discover what works for you.

If you've found this book even a tiny bit helpful, please tell your friends about it, and of course leave me a great review! My mission is to help as many women as possible to get moving, and to enjoy a greater sense of wellbeing as part of a happier, more fulfilled life.

Thank you for taking your first step with me.

If you'd like to continue your journey with my support, I'd love to be there for you. Visit fitbee.co.uk/thelittlebook for the lovely free resources which complement this book. You'll find information on how you can work with me there too.

Taking care of ourselves and our wellbeing has the most wonderful ripple effect, not only touching our own lives, but also those of our friends and families, as well as society in general. I mean, look at me, writing this book because I took the decision to put myself first, and then felt so great about it that I just had to share my experience with the world.

We're all on a journey, so may yours be filled with health, happiness and Active Wellbeing.

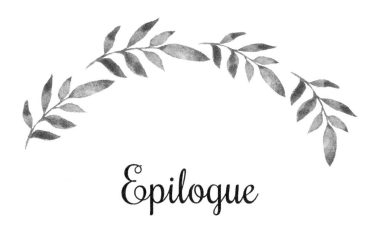

Epilogue

18 November 2020, 2pm

I'm just back in from a walk. I have that warm 'hot flush' feeling you get from coming back inside after being blasted by fresh autumnal air, and to top it off, it's been raining, allowing me to feel totally immersed in the weather as wind, rain and the last of the falling leaves swirled around me.

I have come to love my walks, usually a two-mile trip 'around the block,' which luckily for me includes a short stretch of woodland path – my favourite.

In the past, I often thought about how nice it would be to take regular walks outside, but finding the time always seemed so hard. I would be rushing to work in the car, squeezing meetings into lunch breaks or simply talking myself out of it by looking disappointedly at the weather through the window.

Maybe I'll go later, I'd think, but later never came. There was also a nagging feeling that walking was not 'proper' exercise. *I should be swimming, cycling or running... maybe some weightlifting, too!*

Unfortunately, there were never enough hours in the day.

Then, during the final preparations for the 2017 Edinburgh half-ironman, I had an epiphany. I was at a local race, the Ripon triathlon, and I was jogging around the final 10k run. It was an out and back course, which means that you return on the same route you departed on, and on the way out I passed a man working in his garden.

In that moment, I was struck with envy.

Why was I pushing myself so hard just to go around in circles, not actually getting anywhere except back to the beginning? Meanwhile, here was a man productively immersed in nature. At the end of that day, I would be back where I'd started, whereas he would have a fabulous garden to enjoy.

I had spent months training for the race, for which I would have nothing to show. Yes, the event itself would be great, but the satisfaction is only fleeting. By the next day, or the day after at best, I would have moved on to the next thing. Of course, I had my physical and mental health, and I was in great shape, but I knew that I couldn't sustain my training levels for much longer.

I felt out of balance, in stark contrast to the man kneeling among the flowerbeds, who seemed very much in harmony with his surroundings. He wasn't having to work so hard, either!

These days, I love my walks. I also love soaking up nature, and I love my gardening. I still do some running, yoga and dancing, and although I'd love to eventually get back to open-water swimming (it's lovely once you learn to handle the cold), the most important thing is that I no longer feel stress, pressure or anxiety around exercise. I no longer feel like I must do more. Instead, I do as much, or as little, as I feel like. Enough to feel good.

Am I the fittest I could be? No.

Am I living up to my maximum physical potential? Certainly not.

Do I feel comfortable in my own skin, in balance with life and positive about my choices, knowing that I always have the freedom and opportunity to move my body and feel good? I sure do.

Whatever happens in the future, the knowledge that by simply moving my body, I can come back to myself and feel stronger is a great comfort and energiser. What's more, when so much of the world outside of us seems beyond our control, knowing that I can always nurture and support my internal world through Active Wellbeing is a reassuring thought indeed.

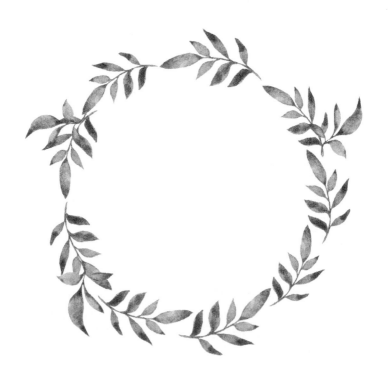

Acknowledgements

There are a few people who I need to thank for helping to make this book happen. First of all, Andrea Morrison, whose amazing coaching first gave me the confidence to take the plunge on this dream project and to keep it going.

I'd also like to thank Gayle Johnson, whose enthusiasm since I first shared my scattered ideas with her has really helped to drive me on. How you organised my rambling thoughts into something coherent remains something of a mystery to me, but I'm very grateful.

My parents, Julie and Gordon Stone, who from an early age instilled in me a belief that I should always go after what I wanted, and that ideas can be made into reality.

Finally, my family, Neal and Oscar, who tolerated the tunnel-focus that it took for me to be able to bring my book into being. For all the piled up dirty dishes, the laundry gathering dust, the missed *Minecraft* games and the bedroom carpet we didn't see for six months, thank you.

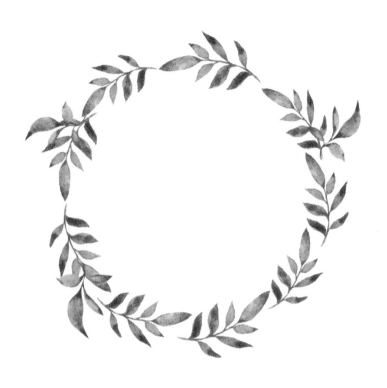

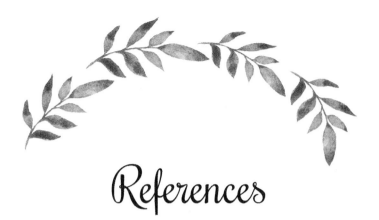

References

1. Cox, E. P. *et al.* Relationship between physical activity and cognitive function in apparently healthy young to middle-aged adults: A systematic review. *Journal of Science and Medicine in Sport* (2016) doi:10.1016/j.jsams.2015.09.003.

2. Chang, Y. K. *et al.* Acute exercise has a general facilitative effect on cognitive function: A combined ERP temporal dynamics and BDNF study. *Psychophysiology* (2017) doi:10.1111/psyp.12784.

3. Kishida, M. & Elavsky, S. Daily physical activity enhances resilient resources for symptom management in middle-aged women. *Health Psychology* (2015) doi:10.1037/hea0000190.

4. Miller, Y. D. & Brown, W. J. Determinants of active leisure for women with young children – An "ethic of care" prevails. *Leisure Sciences* (2005) doi:10.1080/01490400500227308.

5. Lloyd, K. & Little, D. E. Self-determination theory as a framework for understanding women's psychological well-being outcomes from leisure-time physical activity. *Leisure Sciences* (2010) doi:10.1080/01490400.2010.488603.

6. Lloyd, K., O'Brien, W. & Riot, C. Mothers with young children: Caring for the self through the physical activity space. *Leisure Sciences* (2016) doi:10.1080/01490400.2015.1076362.

7. O'Brien, L. Learning outdoors: The forest school approach. *Education 3-13* (2009) doi:10.1080/03004270802291798.

8. Elavsky, S. & McAuley, E. Physical activity and mental health outcomes during menopause: A randomized controlled trial. *Annals of Behavioral Medicine* (2007) doi:10.1007/BF02879894.

9. Sydora, B. C. *et al.* Can walking exercise programs improve health for women in menopause transition and postmenopausal? Findings from a scoping review. *Menopause* (2020) doi:10.1097/gme.0000000000001554.

10. Elavsky, S. Longitudinal examination of the exercise and self-esteem model in middle-aged women. *Journal of Sport and Exercise Psychology* (2010) doi:10.1123/jsep.32.6.862.

11. Teychenne, M. *et al.* Do we need physical activity guidelines for mental health: What does the evidence tell us? *Mental Health and Physical Activity* (2020) doi:10.1016/j.mhpa.2019.100315.

12. Pearson, D. G. & Craig, T. The great outdoors? Exploring the mental health benefits of natural environments. *Frontiers in Psychology* (2014) doi:10.3389/fpsyg.2014.01178.

13. Bragg, R. Nature-based interventions for mental wellbeing and sustainable behaviour: the potential for green care in the UK. *Nature-based interventions for mental wellbeing & sustainable behaviour: the potential for green care in the UK* (2014).

14. Tolle, E. *The Power of Now: A Guide to Spiritual Enlightenment (Book). Library Journal* (2004).

15. Dunstan, D. W., Thorp, A. A., Owen, N. & Neuhaus, M. Sedentary Behaviors and Subsequent Health Outcomes in Adults A Systematic Review of Longitudinal Studies, 1996-2011. *American Journal of Preventive Medicine* (2011).

16. Hausenblas, H. A. & Fallon, E. A. Exercise and body image: A meta-analysis. *Psychology and Health* (2006) doi:10.1080/14768320500105270.

17. UK Chief Medical Officer. UK Chief Medical Officer's Physical Activity Guidelines. *www.gov.uk* 1-66 https://www.gov.uk/government/publications/physical-activity-guidelines-uk-chief-medical-officers-report (2020).

18. Sheeran, P. & Webb, T. L. The Intention–Behavior Gap. *Social and Personality Psychology Compass* (2016) doi:10.1111/spc3.12265.

19. Reyes Fernández, B. *et al.* Action control bridges the planning-behaviour gap: a longitudinal study on physical exercise in young adults. *Psychology and Health* (2015) doi:10.1080/08870446.2015.1006222.

20. Sutton, S. Transtheoretical model of behaviour change. in *Cambridge Handbook of Psychology, Health and Medicine, Second Edition* (2014). doi:10.1017/CBO9780511543579.050.

21. Gerber, J. P., Wheeler, L. & Suls, J. A social comparison theory meta-analysis 60+ years on. *Psychological Bulletin* (2018) doi:10.1037/bul0000127.

22.   Clear, J. Atomic habits: Tiny changes, remarkable results. *Penguin Publicating* (2018).

23.   Steinberg, H. Exercise enhances creativity independently of mood. *British Journal of Sports Medicine* **31**, 240–245 (1997).

24.   Martin, L. *et al.* Nature contact, nature connectedness and associations with health, wellbeing and pro-environmental behaviours. *Journal of Environmental Psychology* **68**, (2020).

25.   Teixeira, P. J., Carraça, E. v., Markland, D., Silva, M. N. & Ryan, R. M. Exercise, physical activity, and self-determination theory: A systematic review. *International Journal of Behavioral Nutrition and Physical Activity* vol. 9 (2012).

26.   Teixeira, P. J., Carraça, E. v., Markland, D., Silva, M. N. & Ryan, R. M. Exercise, physical activity, and self-determination theory: A systematic review. *International Journal of Behavioral Nutrition and Physical Activity* (2012) doi:10.1186/1479-5868-9-78.

Printed in Great Britain
by Amazon